Behavioural Sciences for Dentistry

For Churchill Livingstone:

Commissioning Editor: Michael Parkinson
Project Development Manager: Janice Urquhart
Project Manager: Nancy Arnott
Design direction: Erik Bigland

Behavioural Sciences for Dentistry

Gerry Humphris PhD MClinPsychol
Senior Lecturer in Clinical Psychology,
Department of Clinical Psychology,
School of Health Sciences,
University of Liverpool,
Liverpool, UK

Margaret S. Ling BA(Hons) MA(Econ)
Lecturer in Medical Sociology,
Department of Primary Care,
School of Health Sciences,
University of Liverpool,
Liverpool, UK

Foreword
Anthony S. Blinkhorn BDS MSc PhD FDS
Dean and Clinical Director of the University Dental Hospital of Manchester; Chair of the
Behavioural Sciences in Dentistry Working Group, British Society for Dental Research; and
Executive Committee Member of the Behavioural Sciences and Health Services Research Group of
the International Association for Dental Research.

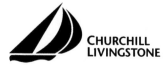
**CHURCHILL
LIVINGSTONE**

EDINBURGH LONDON NEW YORK OXFORD PHILADELPHIA ST LOUIS SYDNEY TORONTO 2000

CHURCHILL LIVINGSTONE
An imprint of Elsevier Limited

First published 2000
  Reprinted 2003, 2004

ISBN 0 443 05190 9

British Library Cataloguing in Publication Data
A catalogue record for this book is available from the
British Library.

Library of Congress Cataloging in Publication Data
A catalog record for this book is available from the Library
of Congress.

Medical knowledge is constantly changing. As new
information becomes available, changes in treatment,
procedures, equipment and the use of drugs become
necessary. The authors and the publishers have, as far as it
is possible, taken care to ensure that the information given
in this text is accurate and up to date. However, readers are
strongly advised to confirm that the information complies
with current legislation and standards of practice.

 your source for books,
journals and multimedia
in the health sciences
www.elsevierhealth.com

Transferred to digital printing 2005
Printed and bound by Antony Rowe Ltd, Eastbourne

Foreword

It can be said with considerable justification that the dental profession has realised that surgical intervention on its own will never solve the problems of dental ill health nor make for satisfied patients. Promoting dental health demands behavioural change and patients' satisfaction with their dentist relates more to efficient communication than to clinical skills.

In the past, successful dentists somehow seemed to learn how to care for the social and psychological problems of their patients. However, for many in the dental profession, there was a disturbing feeling that something was missing from their approach to patient care. Over the last thirty years, behavioural scientists have sought to remedy that deficiency and a number of excellent texts have been produced in an attempt to broaden dentists' perceptions of patient care. Indeed, most dental schools throughout the world have introduced a behavioural science component to the undergraduate curriculum.

Nevertheless, many of these initiatives have been flawed because they have over-emphasised either psychology or sociology, so a balanced view was not presented. It was therefore a delight to read this book 'Behavioural Sciences for Dentistry' by Gerry Humphris and Margaret Ling, which integrates sociology and psychology in such a way that the reader gains a greater insight into the complexities of patient care. The other key feature is that this text is not just a theoretical handbook with little relevance to the practising dentist, it brings problems to life by the inclusion of numerous practical case studies. A revelation and a feature that brings the subject to life with a frisson that is most unusual in texts on psychology and sociology.

So, who will buy this book? Well, practising dentists will find it of great value but dental undergraduates facing all the strain of learning clinical competencies whilst trying to communicate with a patient must read and internalise the advice given by Gerry Humphris and Margaret Ling. They have honed this book on several generations of undergraduates at Liverpool Dental School and as a result the text is clear, precise and highly readable.

I recommend this book to you as a first class aid to patient care, as an introduction to research in an expanding field and as an invigorating read.

Anthony S. Blinkhorn

Preface

Interest in the behavioural sciences is increasing within dentistry. The recent emphasis in dental education on how to present effective messages, encourage patient adherence, improve team working and communication skills indicate several of the areas where behavioural science is making a strong contribution to improving dental health and dental care for patients. This textbook has been written for students studying oral health and is particularly relevant for those who are concerned with patient care. We aim to offer students a basis which will encourage consideration of other influences upon oral health apart from the more traditional approaches adopted by basic sciences such as physiology, biology, biochemistry, immunology and genetics. We hope this text will help you to understand some of the fundamental principles and complexities encountered when working with others, whether they are members of the public or other health professionals. You will find that we have identified the dental practice, engaging the patient, and psychosocial factors connected to oral health, as the major areas in which behavioural science can offer you assistance. We therefore encourage you to read the book as a whole and then to conduct your own projects and enquiries.

Personal pronouns, such as 'he' and 'she' are used interchangeably with no bias intended.

Liverpool
1999

Contents

Introduction

Behavioural science is a relatively new addition to the dental curriculum, and it is widely regarded as an important element for inclusion in dental education. This introductory chapter attempts to define behavioural science and show how learning about this subject will provide overall benefit in practising dentistry and promoting dental care.

To give a single definition of behavioural science that encompasses its many branches is difficult: behavioural science consists of many disciplines that include psychology, sociology and social anthropology, with economics, ethics and communication closely associated. Within all these disciplines one focus tends to be common: each ultimately attempts to explain people's behaviour. The behaviours that are focused upon vary, however. A psychological approach, for example, may examine the fearful reactions of patients to a local anaesthetic injection, whereas the sociological approach may investigate who attends the dentist and offer explanations of why these patients make the decision to seek dental care. The application of economics may focus on the purchasing behaviour of expensive restorative or prosthetic treatments such as implants. Ultimately, behaviour is the common element of interest in all these examples.

Definition of behavioural science in destistry

Behavioural science in dentistry may be defined as the study to understand or explain the behaviour of people in relation to oral health. In order to illustrate why behavioural science has relevance to the dental student this book has been organised into ten further chapters. Each chapter will demonstrate the way in which a behavioural science approach can provide a helpful, perhaps vital ingredient to understanding an aspect of the people whom you will meet in the course of your dental career. The people referred to may be patients, members of the general public or colleagues at work. It is also hoped that the student will appreciate that the methods and theoretical approaches adopted by behavioural science can be a fascinating way of exploring the attitudes, motives and behaviour of those with whom you will be in contact with during your professional life. We believe that gaining an improved knowledge of others, and to some degree of yourself, will assist you as a clinician in how you practise dentistry and consider your influence on the dental health of your locality and the community at large.

In addition, the reader may wish to embark upon an individual project to help answer a question posed by the material in this book. A number of dental organisations – including, for instance, the Faculty of General Dental Practitioners – are encouraging their members to conduct research. This pressure comes from a professional awareness that the knowledge base of dentistry needs expanding. Many of the concerns about dental health focus on the chronic health problems which are a feature of modern Western society: hence the manner in which the dental profession faces the challenges of the future could, potentially, act as an example to other healthcare providers. The application of behavioural sciences is relatively new in the dental field, but the tools of assessment and analysis – a product of these sciences – can assist clinicians in the study of oral health.

Plan of book

This book is divided into three sections:

1. The dental practice: setting the scene (Chapters 2–5)
2. Enabling contact between patient and dental staff (Chapters 6 and 7)
3. Psychosocial factors and oral health (Chapters 8–11).

The adjectives psychological and sociological are often summarised jointly by using the word 'psychosocial'. The first section of this book, comprising Chapters 2–5, concentrates on the centre that provides dental care, in the form of advice and treatment. This has been termed the dental practice and includes the physical location together with all the elements of the service including staff, equipment, philosophy of care and the patients themselves. A single chapter is devoted to each of the following issues:

- Influences on dental attendance. Who visits the dental practice? And why is the decision to attend taken by some people and not others?
- Patients' expectations and their interactions with dentists.
- The dental personnel and changes in the delivery of dental care; the impact of such changes on dental practice staff and on future service provision.

The final chapter of this section considers the social context (setting) of dental care for elderly people. This is a topic of growing importance – in most developed countries, people aged 65 or over now make up an increasing proportion of the total population. Dental care for older people is changing. New materials and techniques make restoration and the design of protheses an option, whereas a decade or so ago such work would not have been possible. The expectations of older patients are changing, and an understanding of these issues may help the clinician predict the way services will be provided to patients of the future.

The second section (Enabling contact: Chapters 6 and 7) focuses on the exchanges between the clinician and the patient. It examines the two major concerns of dental personnel when contacting patients to inform, gain permission to treat or perform treatment procedures, namely communication and dental anxiety. These two areas are also known to be key features of how patients judge their contact with dental personnel. Patients will ask: 'How well did the dental staff members relate to me and how did they manage my nervousness about visiting the dentist?' Included in this section will be some practical suggestions on how to improve communication with certain groups of patients and on reducing levels of fear associated with dental visiting. It is advisable for dental staff to practice some simple precautions to ensure that patients are not driven to seek some form of recompense, through litigation for example. One such method designed to prevent patient complaints is the introduction of informed consent. Working in small teams, as opposed to single-handed practice, is becoming standard, but there are new pressures in the establishment and maintenance of teams. Chapter 10 discusses some barriers to effective team working and how to overcome or prevent them.

The third section (Psychosocial factors and oral health: Chapters 8–11) explores how oral health conditions may be better understood with a working knowledge of behavioural science. In Chapter 8 examples are presented that show how oral health problems are exacerbated by psychosocial factors, and this understanding can assist in the management of these difficulties.

Chapter 9 illustrates how patients will attend dental facilities with psychological problems. Care is needed in their assessment before referral to other appropriate service providers, such as the local hospital or the patient's general medical practitioner. Purchasers of dental services are becoming more sophisticated in their specifications and many are considering general health matters, including psychological care issues.

In Chapter 10 some of the key behavioural science principles that make an important contribution to the dental health promotion field are explained. These principles will assist in the preparation of health advisory messages with an emphasis on the measurable effects on clinical outcomes.

The final chapter provides some background for consideration of the way in which certain programmes can or cannot be evaluated. Resources for embarking on new programmes or even continuing with old, and supposedly established, practices are becoming scarce. A new focus on evidence-based dentistry is questioning current practices using critical approaches that measure what happens with new as well as established treatments, and assess clinical outcomes. Behavioural science has a part to play in assisting the design and implementation of these evaluation projects with the aim of improving oral health. Dental students are expected, as part of their training, to embark on some self-directed project. This is likely to involve the collection and sifting of data (whether collected afresh or archived in a library). An analytical and critical approach to this work will be required and this final chapter will give an overview with recommendations before embarking on such projects.

The use of 'jargon'

Behavioural science is often accused of using a large amount of jargon, and such accusations are not without foundation. All disciplines, however, have their own terminology that provides a shorthand and prevents repetitive explanations. Some of this criticism of behavioural science is therefore a result of unfamiliarity, and the student will need to become conversant with some of the terms that are commonly referred to in the literature. Rather than produce a glossary at the end we have included highlighted boxes which give short definitions of terms that are referred to throughout the text.

A case is presented below which illustrates the need to combine the principles learnt in established courses on oral disease with those of behavioural science.

Case 1a

Sandi, a 15-month-old girl, lives with her 22-year-old mother in a deprived area of the northwest of England. When they visited the health visitor at the local health centre and discussed Sandi's health, one of the questions the child's mother asked was 'When will Sandi be old enough to care for her own teeth?'

The health visitor was surprised by this question because the child's mother had previously discussed Sandi's oral care with her. As a young baby, Sandi's gums had apparently been regularly cleaned using a soft brush dipped in boiled water. However, the mother explained that over the last few months, shortly after Sandi's first birthday, she had stopped brushing the child's gums or new front incisors. When asked her reasons for stopping the regular brushing the mother replied: 'They're only baby teeth and they'll fall out anyway'.

Two alternative explanations of the mother's behaviour may be offered. Had she, perhaps, lost interest in Sandi's oral health? The apparent contradiction between this mother's initial regular care of her child's gums and subsequent lack of concern for the child's deciduous teeth may be accounted for by assuming a sudden loss of interest on the mother's part. Thus, a dentist treating such a child, and relying solely on traditional dental science, would explain the discrepancy between the mother's early behaviour and her statement about her child's deciduous teeth as inconsistent.

A lack of care for deciduous teeth is understood within clinical dental science to be likely to lead to caries which in turn has a damaging effect upon the permanent dentition that follows. It is noted that the brushing of the primary dentition when erupted will not be more resistant to caries unless accompanied by a fluoride-containing dentrifice.

In this case it would be very easy to dismiss this mother's apparently inconsistent behaviour as stemming either from a lack of concern for or a lack of interest in her child's oral health. A consequence of this could be that the dentist might decide any further advice about Sandi's oral health needs would inevitably be disregarded – Sandi would be like so many other children living in deprived areas and would eventually require restorative treatment.

The dentist may of course offer some advice to the mother but it might be coloured by the view that this mother really did not care very much about her child's dental health. Because behavioural science seeks to understand behaviour, there is however an alternative explanation of this behaviour which could be offered and which would improve Sandi's chances of having good oral health, and this explanation is that there was incomplete understanding on the mother's part.

The beliefs people hold about their dental health require understanding. Such lay beliefs are not irrational, and they do not necessarily lack coherence. Further discussion with Sandi's mother supported this. The mother explained that despite her not continuing to help her child brush her own teeth and gums, she was still very interested in her child's overall dental health. The absence of continued care was because she was unaware of the potential for damage to the permanent dentition. In addition, she held a commonsense view regarding her child's deciduous teeth as temporary. A psychosocial approach would allow the mother's understanding and commonsense views to be taken into account, and treatment or advice could be targeted appropriately. The knowledge provided by dental science combined with the understanding offered by behavioural science allows a fuller explanation of the mother's behaviour. A beneficial outcome for her child may result.

Case-based examples

The use of anonymous but real patients in the cases contained in each chapter is intended to provide an interesting and informative context to demonstrate links between theory and practice. The cases also help to prevent the problem of over-generalising. The use of generalisation to indicate widely prevalent common features, usually within large groups of the population, can often provide a valuable overview. However, as case 1a shows, large group generalisations can hide important extreme differences among individuals and small minority groups. The Adult Dental Health Survey of 1988 provides one such example of a series of overviews gathered from a random sample from the adult dentate population of the UK. It describes the dental health of the survey participants. The use of random sampling to select those from whom the information on dental health was gathered enables the findings from the survey to be generalised in order to provide a representation of the state of dental health of the adult population as a whole.

However, when a patient either visits a dentist or decides to become actively responsible for his or her own dental care, very particular or individual experiences, expectations, skills and behaviours are involved. By using real cases it is hoped to demonstrate that people are very diverse and that some helpful insight in explaining human phenomena which otherwise may remain a quirk or oddity, is often better understood when adopting a psychological or sociological approach.

We are confident, therefore, that you will gain from learning some behavioural science and that this process will be of benefit to both you and the patient. It is important, when emphasising the psychosocial aspects of care, that a middle path is established between the person offering the care (frequently referred to as 'the professional') and the person receiving it ('the patient'). The creation of a middle path helps to prevent taking a one-sided view of the provision of dental care. The typical view is associated with the traditional biomedical model, and this regards the patient as a mechanical object without feelings, thoughts, motives, friends or family.

In our description of behavioural science we hope to present a balance between lay (i.e. public) and professional issues. Emphasis will be placed on avoiding the antagonism which often exists between everyday, commonsense and professional approaches. Part of this balance will be presented by stressing the importance of lay health beliefs. If you concentrate on the health beliefs of your patients you are less likely to override their wishes. Patients who are not listened to either withdraw and do not return, or they become overly dependent upon the professional. The cases that are used as the focus for most of the chapters in the book will demonstrate that:

Lay health beliefs are not simply diluted versions of medical knowledge (Nettleton 1995).

These beliefs are vital as they reflect many fundamental areas of a person's life including cultural context, personal biography and social identity. The role of the professionals will also be included when describing psychological and sociological factors associated with dentistry. The dentist will nearly always deliver better dental care, and have greater career satisfaction, if an effort is made to understand patients in some depth (Gift 1977). Therefore advantages have been highlighted for both participants in patient/professional interactions from a knowledge of behavioural science.

The following case example which describes a patient who has good oral health and attends her dentist for regular six-monthly checkups illustrates such a situation.

Case 1b

A young woman of 23 attended a general dental practitioners' (GDP) surgery for a six-monthly checkup. This patient had attended the same dental practice, situated in an affluent suburb of a large city, from early childhood. She first accompanied her parents for their regular checkups when she was young. From the age of one she had been given her own appointment, and had been treated by several different dentists, owing to changes in practice personnel. When she attended a university in the north of England, several hundred miles from home, she still returned for her twice yearly checkup at this practice. She had found general dental practitioners in short supply in the northern town where she attended university.

The young woman had no dental caries, having had her teeth treated with fluoride as a young child, and always used a fluoride toothpaste. She also observed good oral hygiene, a practice which had been encouraged by both her parents. The care had been not only of her permanent dentition, but also of her deciduous teeth. She had therefore never had any restorative dentistry.

This patient and her parents shared similar norms and values about standards of oral health to those of their dental practitioner. (See Box 1.1)

BOX 1.1 DEFINITION OF SOCIAL NORMS AND VALUES

Norms
Rules of conduct which specify appropriate behaviour in a given range of social contexts. A norm either prescribes a given type of behaviour or forbids it.
(Giddens 1997)

Thus the norm in the family (see Case 1a) was to attend the dentist for regular checkups.

Values
Ideas held by human individuals or groups about what is desirable, proper, good or bad.
(Giddens 1997)

This particular family placed emphasis on having good oral health. It was an important aspect of their lives as this young patient's behaviour shows.

Case 1c

At the visit, this patient entered the surgery and after exchanging greetings, sat down facing the dentist, each sitting on hard-backed chairs. The young woman explained that she was shortly moving to live permanently in another part of the country. She would therefore have to find another GDP as soon as she could after moving.

After several minutes discussion about her oral health, the patient moved to sit in the dental chair. She appeared relaxed all the time she was in the dental surgery, even when her teeth were inspected. The dentist commented on the good state of her mouth and her obvious care regarding oral hygiene. The patient then left the surgery, first having thanked the dentist for the care she had received from himself and from the practice over the 20 years she had been a patient.

In this case as the norms and values of the patient and dentist were the same, there was no difference between the need for care identified by the patient (perceived need) and the professionally defined (normative need) which was identified. Such a situation where the perceived and normative needs are the same is not untypical for particular groups of regular dental attenders.

This young woman's norms and values regarding her dental care did not apparently change. At a later date, her mother told this dentist that despite difficulties finding a GDP who was able to accept new patients, her daughter had persisted in her search. She had been successful and was now registered with a dental practice in the area to which she had moved.

The next chapter discusses the issue of dental attendance and considers underlying factors such as the effects of social class groupings on attendance, that is, who attends the dentist. It will also seek to establish why people make the decision to seek treatment.

References

Giddens A 1997 Sociology (3rd edn.). Cambridge: Polity

Gift H 1977 The dental patient's cultural response to the need for dental care. Dental Clinics of North America 23(3): 595–604

Nettleton S 1995 The sociology of health and illness. Cambridge: Polity

PART 1

THE DENTAL PRACTICE: SETTING THE SCENE

2

Attending the dentist

Introduction

One of the most important contributions made by behavioural science to dentistry is its ability to offer understanding of the social factors underlying patterns of oral and dental disease. The aims of this chapter are to:

- Establish who in the population seeks dental care.
- Explore why such people decide to seek professional help.
- Identify the factors and issues that prevent other people obtaining dental care.
- Discover what can turn reluctant patients into loyal practice attenders.

Who seeks care?

An informative and helpful way of investigating who seeks dental care is to consider differences in dental health within the population. Such an approach involves using evidence from social epidemiology which is the study of the distribution of disease, impairment and general health across a population.

Epidemiological information about dental health and disease is available from decennial (ten yearly) national surveys, one of adult dental health and the other of children's dental health. One such UK survey reported on the outcome from dental examination of the mouths of over 4000 adults (Todd & Lader 1991). Data from this survey together with a national survey of children's dental health

(O'Brien 1994) focused upon recording the number of teeth which are decayed, missing or filled (the DMFT Index).

The use of indicators of dental health across generalised and broad social divisions suggests that there are differences in oral health within the population between different social groups. These groups are based upon the concept or category of social class.

What is social class?

Social class is a measure which has been developed within the social and political sciences as a basis for distinguishing social groups according to their status, power, prestige or wealth. Because status is very much concerned with individual views about the way people live and work, for the purposes of epidemiology, this is too subjective an estimate of a person's position within society.

An alternative means of measurement could be to use people's income or wealth, because either seems to be quantifiable in monetary terms. However, the accuracy of such measures has been found to be rather problematic.

Epidemiologists therefore turn to what they regard as more objective (less judgemental) and realisable ways of dividing up the population. Consequently the population is divided into a series of layers each representing different degrees of social and economic power (social stratification). This is a hierarchical distribution of advantage and disadvantage, based upon the perceived priorities of contemporary society. Social stratification therefore describes the pattern of social inequality.

In their analysis of general health inequalities described in the Black Report (Townsend & Davidson 1982), the authors identified social classes as:

'Segments of the population showing broadly similar types and levels of resources ... styles of living ... and some shared perception of their collective condition.' During the twentieth century, the social, cultural and economic characteristics of Britain have created a climate within which, for many purposes, social class can most readily be defined on the basis of occupation.

Social class and occupation

The Registrar General's classification of occupations into five social classes is the index used in national dental surveys; it is normally applied at a household level, determined by the occupation of the head of household, who is usually male. The five occupational groupings are:

Social class	Occupational type
I	Professional
II	Intermediate
III(NM)	Non-manual:skilled non-manual
III(M)	Manual:skilled manual
IV	Partly skilled
V	Unskilled

APPLYING SOCIAL CLASS IN PRACTICE

Two case examples will be discussed in this section of the chapter; one from a general dental practitioner's point of view, the other from a clinical psychologist's account. These two cases illustrate that:

- Stratifying the population into layers that reflect the inequalities between different social groups can provide a useful though somewhat generalised background to the treatment of patients.
- Occupational class provides an awareness of the general differences in oral health that might be expected between the various social classes.
- It is important, when considering an individual's dental care, also to pay attention to his or her particular history and circumstances.

Case 2a   A reluctant attender

This interaction takes place within a general dental practice which comprises two partners, one male and one female, and a female associate, together with a receptionist and three dental surgery assistants (DSAs). The practice is located in an inner suburb of a large industrial town with a mix of housing types and ages and a corresponding mix of social classes and household structures. There is a reasonably convenient public transport service to the dental practice from most parts of the town.

A female patient, aged 25, living in her parents' house with her partner and five-year-old child, visits the dentist. She works part-time in the local supermarket where she began working when she left school at the age of 16.

The female dentist is 30, and is an owner-occupier living with her partner in a house in a more affluent part of the suburb. She has been an associate at this practice since qualifying as a dentist and starting her first job at 23. Unlike the patient – who was born in this town – the dentist comes from a rural area in a different part of the country.

After greeting the patient and asking her about her oral health, the dentist carries out a routine inspection of the patient's mouth. The DSA records the details on her dental chart.

The patient had visited the dentist because she had experienced pain in her mouth. However, she had not had a checkup for between two and three years, and she admitted to feeling slightly ashamed both of her poor attendance and the state of her teeth.

This sense of shame, and vulnerability to perceptions of professional disapproval, were noted in a study by Crawford (1980). Crawford explained how: 'In an increasingly "healthist" culture, health behaviour has become a moral duty and illness an individual moral failing'.

Case 2b, which will be discussed more fully later in this chapter, offers an example of some of the serious consequences patients can face when such feelings of failure become too intense.

Although the patient and dentist in the first case (2a) may be regarded as belonging to different social classes on the basis of their current occupations, the social class of the head of their respective households is not stated here. Indeed, a dentist is rarely aware of such information about a patient's household. The dentist or patient may have a social background rather different from that implied by their current occupation.

However, if the Registrar General's scale were to be applied to this patient, she would probably be classified as in social class III non-manual, which includes shop assistants; whereas the dentist would be regarded as in social class I, professional.

General information, about large sections within the population, such as social class might alert the dentist to predicting whether a patient may be a poor attender. Data in the 1988 National Survey of Adult Dental Health (Todd & Lader 1991) suggests that only 43% of the UK adult dentate population attended regularly for checkups, with a further 14% attending only for occasional checkups, and the remaining 43% visiting the dentist only when they had dental health problems. This survey also indicates that attendance rates are generally lower among social classes III, IV and V.

In this case, however, the dentist planning the patient's treatment sought specific reasons for past poor attendance rather than assuming its inevitability. The dentist was therefore careful to ensure that her own behaviour was not influenced by her perception of the patient's class status.

The dentist discovered that for this particular patient several issues influenced her regular attendance:

- The patient's employment situation.
- The patient's own health beliefs and behaviour.
- The competence gap created by differing patient and dentist norms and values.

The patient's employment situation

Some barriers to attendance and so to care were created by the patient's working hours. Attendance was potentially difficult, because although travel to the dental surgery was easy, she considered the cost of the return fare too expensive. Concern with financial cost was made worse because the patient not only lost earnings through absence from work for things such as dental appointments, she also had to arrange and pay for child care. The patient commented that the provision of child care at the dental practice would be helpful.

When the dentist planned this patient's treatment, she did so with awareness of the problems her patient faced in making repeat visits. While she could do nothing about factors such as the patient's employment, travel arrangements and costs, she decided to raise the issue of child care facilities at the next practice meeting.

The patient's own health beliefs and behaviour

This patient also explained to the dentist that, as the tooth causing her trouble was located in a part of her mouth that was not normally visible, she preferred to have the tooth extracted rather than undergo restorative treatment.

In general, the effect of dental health on personal appearance is of concern to people from all social classes (Reisine 1981). However, where a tooth is not normally visible to others and so personal appearance is not affected, people from social classes III, IV and V tend to place less emphasis on retaining such teeth. In this case, the dentist experienced some difficulty in establishing with the patient the benefits of treating the tooth rather than extracting it.

Apparently, although the patient only had three fillings, her oral hygiene was inadequate and her gums in poor condition, hence the oral pain recently experienced. The dentist spent time explaining the cause of her condition and that the maintenance of healthy gums was as important as taking care of her teeth. She also included advice about diet, emphasising the importance of understanding the role of sugar in caries. The dentist also explained the undesirability of extracting teeth, because although such action solved an immediate difficulty it created future problems with maintaining good health.

THE COMPETENCE GAP: DIFFERING NORMS AND VALUES

Closely linked to this patient's approaches to her dental health are the differing norms (rules) and values (guidelines) evident in the attitudes of the patient and dentist to the appropriate form of treatment. All dental practitioners participate in a process of occupational socialisation which may be described as the way in which the values, attitudes, skills and knowledge are acquired of the culture of which membership is sought. It is therefore necessary, in order to understand the dentist's part in case 2a, to explore some of the meanings that are associated with belonging to the occupational group of dental practitioners. A traditional approach to understanding membership of an occupational group is described by Manson (1994). He argues that dentistry satisfies the criteria of a profession which exists:

> By virtue of methods of selection, long formal education often followed by a long and highly disciplined apprenticeship; as in accountancy and architecture, the law as well as medicine and dentistry, professions become highly exclusive groups which are allowed by law through statutory regulation to monopolise their particular form of activity.

Such an approach as Manson's emphasises the dental practitioner's autonomy, and possession of scientific knowledge (Manson 1994). By possessing such autonomy and knowledge the dental practitioner, as a professional, exercises power over patients. Thus in Case 2a, although social class may indeed play an important part in explaining the different views regarding the appropriate form of treatment for this patient, so does the influence of occupational socialisation.

Tuckett suggests that becoming a professional (i.e. professionalisation) takes place because occupational socialisation ensures that a new entrant is exposed to the predominant norms and values of an occupational group (Tuckett 1982). During the long training period and even during subsequent professional practice, these norms and values are maintained through an informal process of social control by the group.

In Case 2a the patient's remedy for her condition is to have the troublesome tooth extracted, whereas the dentist favours restorative work. These different solutions to the same problem may be explained by different levels of knowledge existing between the dentist and the patient, sometimes referred to as the 'competence gap'.

While such an approach fitted well with the view of the patient depicted in the biomechanical model associated with clinical treatment – where the mind and the body are separate – more recent views have, as Arney and Bergen (1984) described, been concerned with: 'Invoking the presence of the patient, calling him [sic] forward from what once appeared an unbridgeable gulf. It is ending the rule of silence.' Such approaches were embodied in documents focused upon patients and their right to have a voice (Department of Health 1989).

An alternative explanation of how the process of professionalisation operates is suggested by Nettleton (1992). She regards concentration on differences between professional and patient power as unhelpful: 'Dentistry has only been examined in terms of individual or collective power struggles. Writers have seen the growth of a discipline as involving the acquisition of power, this power once grasped can be wielded to the advantage of those who hold it.'

According to Nettleton there has been too much emphasis upon 'diseased mouths': 'It is only by examining ... seemingly trivial practices of everyday life, that we can comprehend the nature and possibility of dentistry.' Such a view of professionalisation emphasises the need for interaction between patients and practitioners which is governed by more equitable and less hierarchical concerns. Perhaps a better description of the desirable type of relationship which should exist between clients and professionals is illustrated by Tuckett (1982). He regards the interaction between dentists and their patients as 'a meeting between experts'. A more detailed view of socialisation is presented in Chapter 3.

OUTCOMES FROM CASE 2a

The patient in this case, although reluctant to accept the dentist's advice, agreed to make two further appointments for restorative treatment. Having attended the first appointment, however, she decided that as she was no longer in pain, she would cancel the second appointment.

When she returned several weeks later because she was experiencing pain in her partially treated tooth, she again made two appointments for treatment. This time she did attend both appointments and completed the course of treatment. One year later she had not attended for any further checkups.

Case 2a has provided some insight regarding who attends the dentist. It illustrates clearly some of the barriers experienced by many patients when seeking dental care. However, whilst both quantitative data on dental attendance and examples such as in Case 1b provide descriptions regarding patterns of attendance and barriers to it, they paint an incomplete picture. To draw a complete and detailed picture it is also necessary to understand why dental care is sought and that some people face even greater barriers because they have had previous unpleasant experiences of dentistry, or even that they are phobic about dentistry.

The following case (2b) explores the way in which an individual's symptoms were perceived, evaluated and acted upon.

Why seek dental care?

This case establishes why – because of the state of his oral and dental health – a 40-year-old male took a series of decisions by which he negotiated his way to seeking professional help.

Case 2b   A patient with dental phobia

This patient was referred to the dental hospital by his general medical practitioner for help in treating his dentition which was in a very serious state, with caries extensively developed in a number of teeth. He had not visited a dentist since childhood (six years of age). The man explained that for many years he had suffered rather a lot of physical discomfort because of his teeth. However, he had become used to the wracking pain which occurred when the nerve of a tooth became exposed as a result of caries, and which often resulted in

an abscess requiring antibiotics. He had lost a number of teeth in this way and some of his remaining teeth were badly discoloured.

This patient was reluctant to seek treatment and was therefore similar to the patient in Case 2a. From this man's own account discomfort or pain alone was not enough to encourage him to seek professional help. As a number of sociologists have suggested, other psychosocial circumstances also have to occur.

Psychosocial influences

Mechanic (1968) described such psychosocial factors as 'variables', Zola (1973) named them 'triggers', whereas Freidson (1970) saw the nature and values of 'lay referral networks' as a major influence on service use. In this particular case, the man went on to explain that not only was he very worried that the sockets which still included the infected roots were going to develop oral cancer, but he had recently become very conscious of the gaps between his teeth. He was very aware that they were noticed by other people.

In their work, Mechanic, Freidson, Zola and more recently Scambler (1991), all emphasise how important cultural and social groups are in illness behaviour. The approach of these social scientists can be used to explain that this patient's decision to seek help may be a result of other factors, apart from either the presence, or the severity, of the symptoms he was experiencing.

Further discussion with the clinical psychologist revealed the extent and complexity of the patient's concern. The patient explained that he had a successful business, working as a plumber, and that after ten years of living alone following a divorce, he had recently begun a new relationship. His new partner was a 38-year-old woman with one child. He now also had a different and much wider circle of friends.

Thus the fact that this patient was involved in new social networks and cultural groups could certainly be a contributory factor with regard to his decision to seek professional help. In his work on 'lay referral networks' Freidson (1970) emphasises the importance of the role of significant others (people who matter to an individual) in illness behaviour.

Among other studies which emphasise the way many patients respond to the meaning rather than the biophysical aspects of their symptoms is work by Kleinman. He focused on the way a person's experience of illness reflects the person's experience of life (Kleinman 1988). He describes how 'illness narrative does not merely reflect illness experience, but rather contributes to the experience of symptoms and suffering'. The patient is thus regarded as a person with a story to tell (that is, their narrative), a particularly appropriate approach to take with a patient such as the man described in the case. His biography incorporates his own beliefs, values and culture. In the medical literature much of the work incorporating such an approach refers to chronic illness (Williams & Calnan 1996). Many oral diseases are chronic in nature. Hence the approach of listening to the person's 'story' of their 'illness' makes it particularly relevant and pertinent to the dental context. Some of the techniques for utilising such an approach are discussed in Chapter 6.

The clinical psychologist probed further after establishing why the patient had decided to seek professional help at that particular time. He asked why such a length of time had elapsed since the man had sought any professional dental care. The reply was very revealing and led to a diagnosis that the patient was phobic about dentistry following a traumatic incident when receiving general anaesthesia at the age of six.

The man was seen by the clinical psychologist in the dental hospital but in a non-dental clinical environment (that is, an office with two comfortable chairs and a coffee table). He showed clear physiological signs of anxiety with profuse perspiration from the forehead and hands, and complained of stomach cramps. He appeared agitated and fidgeted in his chair. He was very intense in his manner and alert to noises outside the consulting room, such as the muffled slamming of a door. He reported being close to panic in reporting his difficulties but eventually reduced his anxiety level when it was explained to him repeatedly that he would not be receiving any

examination or treatment on this or the next couple of visits, neither would he be introduced to a dentist.

> After such reassurance, the patient went on to relate his experience in extensive detail including a description of the dentist and the building in which he received the treatment. He found the experience very distressing, remembering vividly his dream following the removal of his tooth.
>
> He reported that he saw himself swimming in a pool of blood and had woken up experiencing confusion, with some pain and nausea and sockets which bled. He had not attended the dentist again prior to his visit to the dental hospital to see the clinical psychologist.

This patient's dental disease offered little interference with his usual everyday social activities, and therefore he did not seek treatment. It was only when his oral condition promoted repeated acute symptoms (pain), caused the patient to fear the development of a serious condition such as oral cancer, and comments about the appearance of his teeth were made by significant others, that he took the decision to seek professional help.

More barriers to care

Awareness of the social factors related to disease are again particularly important when – as the patient in the case above shows – there are significant barriers to seeking treatment. This patient, when discussing his reluctance to seek treatment with a clinical psychologist, and despite the painful state of his mouth, recalled what he termed a 'vivid dental experience' when he was six years old.

Accounts of similar vivid experiences were recorded by just under a quarter of adults participating in the 1988 survey (Todd & Lader 1991). The patient in this case was within the age range of dentate adults aged 35–44 whose vivid dental experience occurred under the age of 16 and involved gas.

In a study by Finch (1988), similar experiences to those of this patient were reported by participants who recalled childhood experiences of having gas. These people, like this patient, considered the vivid experience to have created a barrier to their seeking dental care in adulthood. Such barriers are then incorporated within the patient's subsequent behaviour and attitudes to dental care. As this particular case shows, even in the presence of what must have been increasingly evident signs and symptoms, it was a long time before this patient sought professional help or advice.

OUTCOMES FROM CASE 2b

After a series of visits (six at weekly intervals) the patient was able to enter a dental surgery. He underwent some treatment under sedation but had continuing and significant problems attending the dentist. He was fortunate in that as well as clinical help from the members of the dental team, he also received continuing support from his partner.

Having established who attends the dentist and discussed the underlying rationale for attendance, the remaining section of this chapter will be used to outline some ways in which dental practitioners can help to break down barriers to seeking care.

Non-attender to loyal patient

The case below (2c) briefly demonstrates that barriers to attending the dentist can be broken down by preliminary encounters (such as accompanying a child). The effect upon the potential patient of such a chance encounter will depend upon how the staff of the practice as a whole present to the patient as well as the appearance of the practice.

The concern of the rest of this chapter is to outline some of the factors which determine whether patients will remain with a practice or wish to move on.

There are some important variations in the degree of loyalty to visiting the same dentist over time, as shown in the Adult Dental Survey (Todd & Lader 1991). The benefits to the dentist of keeping their patients include completion of the course of

---

Case 2c Dental practice and patient loyalty

A woman in her 30s who was a non-attender, reported in discussion with one of the authors that 'I would not have set foot in a dental practice until I went with my son to have his teeth checked. I was surprised how much dentists had changed as the place looked welcoming and the staff were prepared to chat.' She continued by saying that her concerns centred on general fears including how much work was needed on her teeth and gums and what it would cost. The practice she visited with her son was ready to discuss these worries with her. She therefore began to trust the practice personnel to advise her and give her information on her dental health status and on how to improve her dental health.

---

treatment, fewer case sheets to store (either on card or electronic media), reduced need for extended advertisement to attract new patients and therefore reduced need for lengthy initial interviews to learn about a patient's history and concerns. The advantages for the patient of remaining with a dentist over time include the continuity of care which the dentist can provide: for instance, carious lessions may be left for the next checkup to determine if restoration is required. With a greater mobility in the employment market there is, however, an increasing likelihood of patients moving on to different areas. The Adult Dental Survey reflected that 70% of patients who had lived for less than ten years in the same area compared with 84% who had lived more than ten years claim they would continue visiting the dentist as they did previously. Eighty-two per cent of UK dentate adults said they would attend the same dentist, thereby leaving 18% who expected to change their dental practice the next time they visited the dentist. Those dentate adults who mentioned that they were going to change dentist stated that the reason for doing so was that it was no longer convenient. Unfortunately this does not identify what could be a variety of reasons for their stated inconvenience. Seventeen per cent of participants in this survey were dissatisfied with the dental treatment they had received. They intended to select another practice. It was not clear from the survey in what specific way the treatment had not been to the patients' satisfaction. Reasons may include technical problems encountered during the treatment procedure, patient pain and discomfort or possibly lack of explanation.

Ten per cent of patients disliked the dentist personally. There were some clear sex differences. Dentate women were significantly more likely to say that they were dissatisfied with their dental treatment (19% compared with 15%) or to dislike their dentist (14% compared with 7%) but there was little variation in these two reasons by occupational background. The strength of the dentist–patient relationship, which will be referred to in the next chapter, is considered important in explaining loyalty to a dentist. Respondents to a survey in Florida, USA did not return to their dentist within a five-year span because, in the main, the communication between dentist and patient was poor (Collett 1969). Patients evaluate their dentists with reference to three main factors: Information – Communication, Understanding – Acceptance and Technical Competence (Corah, O'Shea & Bissell 1985). These factors were identified by clustering together mathematically, using a procedure known as principal components analysis, question responses from a detailed survey of patient dental satisfaction. Hamilton and Rouse (1991) propose that patients prefer their dentists to share information and comfort. With the exception of assessing technical competence, which a member of the public is unable to do accurately, it appears that two features are predominant in selecting and maintaining loyalty to a clinician: information giving and emotional support (Nichols 1993).

A recent study (Holt & McHugh 1997) specifically asked regularly attending patients in England and Wales why they chose to stay with their particular dentist or dental practice. The study quoted 'care and attention', 'pain control', 'dentist putting you at ease', 'safety conscious' and 'explanation of treatments' as the highest priority factors. These five aspects reflect the dentist's behaviour and personal skills in relating to patients. However it would be interesting to investigate further patients' views of what constitutes 'care and attention'.

Conclusion

Although it is very easy to place all patients who fail to attend for dental treatment in one category as non-attenders, such a broad generalisation contributes little to an understanding of why this should be so. The use of the cases in this chapter has indicated that it is possible to establish not only who does not attend the dentist, but also to be aware of the variety of factors, that can influence dental attendance.

While it is appropriate to be aware of inequalities in dental health, it is equally important that dental practitioners who treat patients avoid the use of such divisions to create stereotypes (rigid and inflexible categories). Rigid inflexible categorisation (stereotyping) is unhelpful when attempting to treat individual patients. This is particularly so regarding reluctant patients who have plucked up courage to attend. These general categories should be used in conjunction with an individual patient's requirements to help create loyal practice attenders.

References

Arney W, Bergen B 1984 Medicine and the Management of Living. Chicago: Chicago University Press

Collett H 1969 Influence of dentist–patient relationship on attitudes and adjustment to dental treatment. Journal of the American Dental Association 79(4):879–884

Corah N, O'Shea R, Bissell G 1985 The dentist–patient relationship: perceptions by patients of dentist behaviour in relation to satisfaction and anxiety. Journal of the American Dental Association 111:433–446

Crawford R 1980 Healthism and medicalisation of everyday life. International Journal of Health Services 10:365–368

Finch E 1988 Barriers to the receipt of dental care. London: Social and Community Planning Research

Freidson E 1970 The profession of medicine: A study of the sociology of applied knowledge. New York: Harper Row

Department of Health 1989 Working for patients. London: HMSO

Holt V, McHugh K 1997 Factors influencing patient loyalty to the dentist and dental practice. British Dental Journal 183:365–370

Kleinman A 1988 The illness narratives: suffering, healing and the human condition. New York: Basic Books

Manson J 1994 Some problems of professionalism today. British Dental Journal 176: 290–294

Mechanic D 1968 Medical Sociology. London: Free Press

Nettleton S 1992 Power, pain and dentistry. Milton Keynes: Open University Press

Nichols K A 1993 Psychological care in physical illness (2nd edn.) London: Chapman & Hall

O'Brien M 1994 Children's dental health: United Kingdom 1993. OPCS Social Survey Division. London: HMSO

Reisine S 1981 Theoretical considerations in formulating sociodental indicators. Social Science and Medicine 15A:745–750

Rouse R, Hamilton M 1991 Dentists evaluate their patients: an empirical investigation of preferences. Journal of Behavioural Medicine 14(6):637–648

Scambler G (ed.) 1991 Sociology as applied to medicine. London: Balliere Tindall

Todd J E, Lader D 1991 Adult dental health: United Kingdom 1988. OPCS Survey Division. London: HMSO

Townsend P, Davidson N 1982 Inequalities in health: the Black report. London: Penguin

Tuckett D 1982 Introduction to medical sociology. London: Tavistock

Williams S, Calnan M (eds.) 1996 Modern medicine: Lay perspectives and experiences. London: UCL Press

Zola I K 1973 Pathways to the doctor: From person to patient. Social Science and Medicine 7:677–689

3

Expectations of the consultation

When patients visit a dental practice they arrive with expectations about the treatment and care they hope to receive. However, as Lahti et al. (1996) indicate, there is little research focusing on patients' expectations of an 'ideal dentist'. More is known about professionals' expectations of patients (e.g. Morgan 1991).

When patients and dentists meet in the dental surgery their mutual expectations are superseded by a shared experience which may confirm and reinforce these expectations or may be contrary to them in either a positive or negative way. It must be appreciated that although the experience of patient and dentist within a consultation is jointly shared, their perceptions of the interaction may be very different. Both dentist and patient perceive the experience in the light of their previous expectations. It is therefore important to understand both patients' and dentists' expectations of each other and of the dental consultation. These expectations, and patterns of attendance, shape the dental experience thus modifying future expectations.

An insight of expectations can be achieved either through the study of individual cases or by adopting a more generalised approach which considers different models of the dentist–patient interaction. To gain insight into some of the factors which can influence both the patient's and dentist's expectations of each other, two cases are used for illustration. These cases will explore:

- How the individuals involved take part in social processes through which they develop an awareness of norms and values underlying the parts they play as either patient or dentist (socialisation).

- Characteristics or models of the interaction between patients and dentists.

Case 3a Patient expectations met with minimal intervention

Gender: Female   Age: 35   Occupation: Primary school teacher

Referral: Secondary referral from consultant in restorative care

Problem: Fear of amalgam

Features: Strong desire to have amalgam fillings replaced

This woman was seen for a single session by the clinical psychologist. She had been referred because she was considered obsessional about her desire to have all her amalgam fillings removed and replaced with 'white' filling material. She was not convinced that the explanations supplied by the dentist were correct and she agreed to see someone (a clinical psychologist) at the dental school to discuss her fear of having amalgam in her mouth. The clinical psychologist listened carefully to the wishes that the patient expressed about the treatment she requested. She did not regard her views as obsessional and took exception to being regarded as someone with extreme views. The patient was asked how she felt about having to come to the dental school and discuss her concerns. She explained that she thought there was a potential deception being adopted and she

---

wished to gain an ally to convince the dental staff at her local surgery to carry out the treatment she wanted. The patient was encouraged to express her feelings about the possible side effects of mercury amalgam. She was asked to outline the evidence she drew on from past experiences and information from magazines and television. It was of particular importance to ask her for personal instances which were indicative of the harm she felt the amalgam must be doing to her health. Simple closed questions were adopted to focus on instances that led her to believe in the harm for which amalgam must be responsible. The clinician attempted some explanation with the caution that there was still not enough information to be able to make categorical statements that amalgam was completely harmless (Eley 1998). The practice of summarising what the patient has said in the session, of reflecting the patient's emotional reactions and checking with her that she had been able to express her concerns accurately led the patient to reconsider her request. The patient stated that having someone take her worries seriously was enough to ensure that she had been heard properly. This was very satisfying for the patient and made her reconsider insisting on extensive amalgam replacement. She did revisit her dental surgery and asked for a small number of replacement fillings to restore a satisfactory appearance.

Case 3b   Patient expectations unfulfilled

Gender: Female   Age: 40   Occupation:
                                        Housewife
Referral: Secondary referral from consultant in prosthetics
Problem: Low sense of self-worth and low self-esteem
Features: Believed teeth to be discoloured yellow and consequently felt socially embarrassed and inadequate

This woman was convinced that her teeth were yellow and needed to be crowned to restore them to a white and pristine finish. She was seen on two occasions. The same procedures adopted in Case 3a were employed and a history of self-consciousness and lack of social confidence were found. The woman described how, when she was 12, a dentist had said that her teeth were 'dirty' and that she needed to clean them regularly. She was very upset by this, not having been aware that her teeth were in any way discoloured. Objective assessment by the dentist showed normal colouration for the age of the woman's teeth although they were definitely yellowish in appearance. The woman did not smile, and this gave her a wooden, unanimated facial expression. She became very upset when expressing her distress at never being happy with her teeth and how it has affected her social interactions throughout her life. This more severe and fixed belief was not influenced greatly by the use of communication skills as outlined, however the patient did feel as if someone had listened and understood her long-term predicament. She did accept a further dental examination but only with a view to negotiating the possible covering of her discoloured teeth with some of the new materials available.

The first case (3a) showed that the patient eventually had her expectations met. The second case however remained unresolved. The patient continued to press for the treatment she wanted to be provided. This in her eyes was an acceptable dental appearance. This chapter will therefore explore in the first instance socialisation, and secondly, that when patients and professionals do interact, there are often difficulties in meeting patient expectations.

Socialisation

A contributory factor to each of these women's unrealised expectations about their dental care could be the different types of socialisation they experienced and those experienced by members of the dental healthcare team. In addition to their 'everyday socialisation', the professionals had also participated in 'occupational socialisation', a process which involves acquiring the values, norms, attitudes and knowledge of the professional culture to which they belong (see Chapter 2).

Socialisation is important in determining the values and attitudes of both dentists and patients, and there are several different views on how socialisation operates. Examination of these views will help give an insight into the role of socialisation in how people learn to become dentists and how to act as patients. It will also provide an indication of the scope of sociology in providing an understanding of aspects of dental practice.

DIFFERENT APPROACHES TO SOCIALISATION

A distinction was made by Cooley (1902) between two stages of socialisation:

- **Primary socialisation** is characterised by the personal closeness of its contact, usually occurring within families, childhood peer groups and in neighbourhoods;
- **Secondary socialisation** which is more imper-sonal, taking place in schools, colleges or other educational establishments and at work, with individual concerns focused on long-term goals and aspirations.

NORMS AND VALUES

This description of socialisation offers an example of the *consensus structuralist* perspective in sociology, a perspective or guideline that focuses upon the importance of maintaining all the parts or institutions of society in a state of equilibrium or balance. Parsons belongs to this group of sociologists and so uses the primary/secondary distinction to explain how societal norms (rules) and values (general guidelines) are learnt by individuals at the appropriate stage of their development (Parsons 1951). Rules and guidelines (norms and values) are seen as not only having to be learnt correctly, in keeping with the needs of the social system, but

also as having to be learnt at an appropriate time. This connection between what was learnt by a member of society and the time at which the learning occurs, was regarded by Parsons as being of particular importance in order to ensure that any social system was able to function and run smoothly.

Example to illustrate consensus structuralist perspective

A young person leaving school and beginning to train as a dentist will be directed into a strict and highly ordered system of learning. For patients to be able to accept other people having access to their mouths to exercise treatments, society supports an organised structure of a dental school based within a university with all its attendant regulations and links with professional bodies.

A consequence of Parsons' approach is that the person is regarded as passive, as something fashioned and shaped by societal requirements. The person may be likened to a puppet with society pulling the strings to make the puppet function in accordance with societal needs and expectations. Applying such an approach to Cases 3a and 3b would therefore involve placing great emphasis on the wider environment of the patients (sometimes referred to as the 'macro' environment). A relevant example would be how oral health behaviour has been shaped by the norms of a lifestyle which generally applies within the patient's social environment. Primary socialisation is believed to be responsible to a great degree in the formation of a child's dental behaviour, especially toothbrushing (Grytten et al. 1988).

This view of socialisation highlights three things, namely convention, conformity and the social environment within which individuals are directed. It is important to recognise that patients and professionals are considered to be almost totally directed in their actions. There is very little room for people to be diverted in their roles. The behaviour of both the patient and the professional is determined by the society in which they find themselves, and this is known as social determinism. The implication of this view is that any differences between these groups, that is patients and professionals, is seen almost as inevitable and therefore little change is possible. In other words the differences between these groups is irreconcilable.

In Case 3a and 3b, the gap between the women's knowledge and the professional or expert knowledge of the dental team is responsible for there being an irreconcilable difference. The term 'competence gap' is used to describe such a difference. The gap arises because the period of secondary socialisation has – for the dentists – not only been extended, but has also involved highly specialised training. To a lesser extent this is true for other members of the dental teams.

This rigid categorisation of socialisation into primary and secondary stages is, however, inappropriate for practical purposes. Most people acquire their norms and values in a whole variety of places and settings, and over varying stages of their lives. If such a formal and fixed process of socialisation were in evidence then the work to attempt change in people's behaviour (either patient or professional) would be redundant. Therefore other approaches to understanding the socialisation process are worth considering.

INDIVIDUALS, CREATIVITY AND NEGOTIATION

An alternative view of socialisation regards human beings as creative and active participants, who in any social setting are involved in negotiating their roles. This is known as the *interactionist* perspective, and the process of socialisation operates as follows:

- Socialisation begins in early childhood, with the *play stage* in which children adopt roles and play 'let's pretend'. They do this through interacting with *significant others* (people who are important to them).
- These children subsequently engage in the *game stage* which involves interaction with *generalised others* (the collective viewpoint of the others playing in the game).

Such children therefore only have the potential for becoming integrated within society, when they are able to engage with generalised others. This 'taking the role of the other' is a central focus of social interaction (Mead 1934). It is by role-taking that the individual develops a concept of 'self'.

'The role of the other'

Assuming this role involves the following process:

- Reflecting on one's own self and behaviour;
- Undertaking such reflection from what is imagined to be the viewpoint of another; and
- Anticipating the other's reaction.

Such observation is possible as the individual self is divided into two parts, the 'I' and the 'me'. The 'I' engages in the self-observation and reflection, adapting and arranging behaviour in the light of this assessment. Thus a concern with personal appearance, as exhibited by the women in both cases cited above, illustrates how the face, mouth and teeth can reflect the self or inner awareness and the body which houses social obligations and provides a focus for others' comments.

This view of socialisation therefore suggests that the individual is more self-directed than is implied by the passive approach of Parsons. The individual actively creates and shapes the social environment within which interaction takes place. For instance in Case 3b the woman had a clear view of what colour her teeth should be and was actively impressing her view on the dental personnel she saw. Hence the difference between the woman's (lay) and the dentist's (professional) norms and values would be viewed as an example of each participant (patient and dentist) having different meanings over what was an acceptable tooth colour. As the participants in any interaction are constantly negotiating and renegotiating their roles, both the professionals and the patients could be regarded as 'experts'. This is an important idea as only the dentist may be considered 'the expert' in this working relationship. Patients are expert in a number of ways including, for instance, their own physical and emotional sensations, and their perception of the services they use. The notion that both patients and dentists can be considered as experts is possible because of the flexibility of the way roles are developed within the interactionist approach, and in which roles are constructed rather than imposed.

Such an approach as the interactionist one described above, unlike consensus structuralism, does not dismiss individuality as unimportant and so would certainly encourage the dentist in either of the cases not to dismiss the women merely as non-compliant, or non-adherent to professional advice. This not the full story however. The manner of how individuals make sense of their environment and create their own sense of reality is also dependent on their own sense of self-consciousness. The individual, not only turns to culture but also uses her own self-consciousness as a reference point when analysing and assessing situations to create her own sense of reality (Cohen 1994). Box 3.1 summarises the different ways of understanding socialisation by including some dental examples.

Realisation that a person may draw upon individual consciousness when engaging in any social process, such as the process of socialisation, can provide important insights, particularly with regard to interpreting the behaviour of the two women described in Cases 3a and 3b. This is particularly so because the interactionist perspective grounds socialisation within the individual's immediate environment (i.e. microenvironment). In addition, this perspective is an ongoing process rather than a series of defined stages. Finally, people are involved as active participants in such a process. Thus, a patient's oral health may indeed be subject to influences outside the control of the dental team – for example, she may exist on a low income with all its attendant problems. So whereas patient expectations and responses may have been conditioned to some extent by their past socialisation, there is room for individual response. These women, unlike many other non-compliant or non-adherent patients, were particularly concerned about their oral health. Their concerns gave rise to expectations regarding dental treatment which were, not however, shared by the dental professionals.

As the cases indicate, attempting to resolve such differences inevitably involves the establishment of a dialogue between the patient and the dental practitioner, either directly or through the mediating activities of the clinical psychologist.

Whilst the examples quoted in the two cases are in some respects somewhat extreme, many patients hold rather different expectations regarding their dental treatment and the role of the dentist, than are held by dental practitioners. Such differences are highlighted in a Finnish study (Lahti et al.

BOX 3.1	DIFFERENT APPROACHES TO SOCIALISATION	
Description	*Dental example*	*Sociologist*
Fixed and dependent on broad environmental factors	Diet – and therefore sugary snacks – can be considered to be strongly dependent on a fixed socialisation process, making change very difficult.	Parsons
Some flexibility of outcome due to individual entering into an interaction with others	Individual who requires a full denture may consult others, such as spouse and family, over preference on aesthetics of denture and present a request to dentist for a particular finished result.	Mead
A very flexible system where individuals refer to their own norms and values frequently and enter into constant dialogue and negotiation	An individual who wishes to be given implants rather than have a removable prosthesis. Individual makes reference to his or her own values of retaining a permanent and fixed dentition. Discusses requirement with implantologist over shape and colour of tooth.	Cohen

1996b), which found that despite differences in many of their expectations of each other, both dentists and patients held a common view regarding the importance of mutual communication. It is therefore appropriate, to consider next another aspect of the microenvironment of patients and dentists – the patient–dentist interaction.

The patient–dentist interaction

The cases included in this and indeed in all the other chapters of this book, convey the importance of the interaction that takes place between professionals and clients. Such an interaction can have implications, not only for the communication that takes place within it, but also for the influence it exerts on the outcome of care. In this chapter the focus of the patient–dentist interaction will therefore be approached from a microperspective: this includes such topics as class, and so inevitably has an effect upon this interaction. (See Chapter 2 for a fuller discussion.)

THE STYLE OF THE INTERACTION

The two women patients in the cases presented in this chapter, both, as we have seen, exhibited a great deal of concern about their dental health. However, each of these women provides an example of unsuccessful interaction between herself and the dental practitioner.

Individual preferences

In Case 3a the woman patient explained that she was unsure about the accuracy of the information she had received both from the dental practitioner and from the practice staff. Her discomfort was intensified when she found herself labelled as 'extreme', because she had been unable to gain the information she required to allay her fears of having amalgam fillings in her mouth.

In the second case, the patient reported unpleasantness in the way information was given to her by a dental practitioner. Although this had occurred when she was 12 years old – over 25 years earlier – the impact of such an event upon the woman had been substantial, affecting her attitudes and behaviour in many ways and continuing into her adult life. Lack of care in explaining aspects of her dental state in an appropriate manner had not only prevented the effective transmission of information to the patient, it had also resulted in misinformation which caused ongoing and extreme distress.

Appropriate interaction between the patient and the dentist is important not only in respect of restorative dentistry, but is vital in achieving effective preventive care. A study by Croucher (1989) that discussed patient–dentist interaction and the use of preventive strategies in periodontal disease, suggested that many patients considered the information that they were given personally irrelevant.

RELEVANT INFORMATION

Making information relevant to the individual receiving it obviously involves an appreciation of their particular circumstances and their individual needs and preferences. The importance of the dentist ensuring that interaction with patients takes account of different individual preferences was reported by Green, Lang and Jacobson (1988) in a study which discussed how patients had preferences for certain behaviours adopted by dentists. An example of one such issue was the use of formal or informal modes of address. The study reported that 80% of patients preferred to be addressed in an informal way, irrespective of the dentist's age or gender; however, women and older patients generally preferred more formal modes of address. The study lists several other patient preferences, including the use of handshaking, eye contact and introductions between patients and dental staff.

All these examples convey the diversity present among patients, which supports the earlier discussion regarding the importance of the individual and individual consciousness. For the purposes of clarity in discussion, however, it is sometimes necessary to think in categories and to use these categories to aid explanation. The rest of this chapter will therefore discuss some of these different categories or models, in order to help understand the nature of the interaction between patients and their dentists.

MODELS OF PATIENT–DENTIST INTERACTIONS

It has already been established that the way in which patients and dental personnel relate to each other is complex. Sociological approaches already presented have expressed that there are influences from the way in which individuals are brought up, i.e. the phenomenon of socialisation. A further method of examining the relationship between patient and dentist is to apply some of the models of patient–clinician interactions that have been applied mainly to medical situations. These models can, with good effect, help us understand some of the difficulties that may be experienced by patient and dentist.

The interaction that occurred in each of the Cases 3a and 3b included participation by both the women and the professional. The professional made clear his interest in what the women had to say, as well as actively inviting their participation in the interaction. In both cases, the women considered the outcome of this consultation to have been more positive than the encounters they had previously experienced with their dental practitioners. This more successful outcome from the consultation with the clinical psychologist may be explained, albeit simplistically, by the adoption of a psychosocial rather than a biomechanical model.

Because human social interaction is complex, there are various models of patient–professional interaction. The cases presented in the chapter will therefore be discussed from the point of view of four models of patient professional interaction as presented in Box 3.2.

BOX 3.2	DIFFERENT MODELS OF PATIENT–DENTIST RELATIONSHIP
Name of model	*Essential features*
Consensus	Individual takes on a 'sick role'. This enables individual to shun social responsibilities but requires dentist to acknowledge that individual has serious 'disease'. *Example*: Patient with raging toothache.
Mutual dependence	Three different types of relationship which vary according to the degree of participation of the dentist in understanding the patient's predicament. *Example*: Dentist actively sets out to discover reasons for a patient's insistence on having all amalgam fillings removed and replaced with 'white' fillings.
Conflict	Model assumes that patient–dentist interaction is really a conflict relationship and not one characterised as a mutual participation of assessing each other's requirements from the working relationship. *Example*: Dentist wishing to supply a standard and acceptable treatment (i.e. amalgam restorations) that the patient is unhappy to receive.
Conflict and control relationship	Model assumes variation in control. *Example*: Dentist adopts different styles of interactions. The different approaches adopted take account of the patient's characteristics and dental health problems.

Model 1: Consensus

The 'sick role' highlighted how illness not only has a biological form, but also a social one (Parsons 1951). Thus the experience of sickness is concerned with more than the onset of symptoms and of disease. The sick role is a way of controlling social deviance, which unlike criminal deviance, is not seen as the individual's responsibility, although it prevents the fulfilment of an individual's social roles. Access to the sick role requires the sanction of a gatekeeper, who within the biomedical model is the doctor. An example may be a patient who believes that their jaw is abnormally wide and looks disfigured. The perception of an abnormality by the patient requires sanction by a maxillofacial surgeon. The patient may take on a sick role which enables them to bypass their social responsibilities (such as continuing to go to work).

There has been discussion within the literature (Davis 1976; Petersen 1990; Reisine 1981) regarding the relevance of the sick role to dentistry. It has been suggested that this model is more suited to acute rather than to chronic forms of illness. Being acutely ill (for example, raging toothache) provides certain privileges which permit exemption from everyday obligations such as going to work, and responsibility for the illness may be deferred or ignored completely. Demands requiring the patient to seek care and to get well are a feature of the sick role. However, the cases in this chapter show that the assumption of the sick role may well have been appropriate for each of the patients concerned, such was the intensity of their experience and the consequent severity of their symptoms. Such an individual can behave as a social deviant (i.e. stay off work, rely on others to do errands and duties, become irritable) as long as he or she, as a patient, takes on a sick role. The patient can behave in a very passive manner, and this suits the authoritative role of the professional. These distortions of personal behaviour – both from the patient and the clinician – can exist during the patient–dentist interaction.

Model 2: Mutual dependence

Szasz and Hollender (1956) developed Parsons' consensus model further. They described three basic models of the 'physician–patient' relationship, linking them to the patient's illness experience:

- Activity–passivity related to patients who could not actively participate because they were either unconscious or incapable.
- Guidance–co-operation related to forms of acute illness.
- Mutual participation related to forms of chronic illness.

Ayer (1982) suggested that such ways of understanding patient–clinician interactions are applicable to dentistry, and indeed the cases presented in this chapter are usefully described by using them. Both of the cases could be described as fitting within the first of Szasz and Hollender's models. The patients in both cases were somewhat passive and the dentists were reluctant to agree to the demands they placed upon them. However the patients were obviously not incapable either physically or in their ability to persuade. Different ways of construing the patient–dentist interaction are needed (see Chapter 6). The second model is more appropriate to aspects of the consultations with the clinical psychologist rather than with the dentists, since that model allows for an interaction which is characterised by a patient who is adherent because value is placed upon the professional advice which is regarded as a form of expertise. Thus each patient takes account of the advice offered, with each woman balancing her own preferences with the advice she is given by the clinical psychologist.

There are problems in applying this model to dentistry, because so many oral conditions are chronic in nature, but manifest as episodic bouts of acute pain or discomfort. This is perhaps what has taken place regarding the patient in the first case. Her fillings have been in place for some time, but her response to their presence has been fuelled by her concern about amalgam.

The third model, which emphasises the inclusion of both individual preferences and relevant information during the interaction to help ensure patient satisfaction, is particularly appropriate to the interaction with the clinical psychologist described in the first case. In this case, because the patient considered she had been offered advice which not only was relevant to her individual needs, but also supplied the information she sought about the amalgam, was able to be helped by the professional to help herself.

Model 3: Conflict

Freidson (1970) commented that he observed within the doctor and patient interaction a marked degree of conflict, which was certainly evident within the descriptions of the cases of the two women's interactions with their dentists. He based his critique upon a rejection of the assumption that the professional was always active and the patient always passive. The cases presented in this chapter clearly support such a view. Freidson also drew attention to the effect on the interaction that divergence in cultural background of the professional and patient might have.

More recent developments in behavioural science theory have sought to draw upon the two separate traditions of consensus and conflict represented by Szasz and Hollender (1956) and Freidson (1970) respectively and to combine these two approaches. This has resulted in the development of Stewart and Roter's model of patient–professional interaction.

Model 4: Conflict and control

A model which takes account of cultural and other factors such as the stage and type of illness is found in a more recent view of interaction presented by Stewart and Roter (1989). Their model offers four different types of relationship: paternalistic, mutualistic, consumerist and default.

Regarding the patients described in the cases, both women were subjected to a paternalistic relationship. In this type of relationship emphasis is placed upon high professional and low patient control. A clear correspondence exists between this approach and Parsons' depiction of the 'sick role'. As the situation of the women patients involved in interactions with their dentists shows, much onus in terms of decision making was placed upon the dentists. The patients were also expected to place great reliance upon the dentist, so highlighting their passivity.

Mutuality is the aspect of Stewart and Roter's model which is particularly important when attempting to meet both dentist and patient expectations. Mutuality highlights the value of diminishing conflict by apportioning equal control to both patient and professional within the interaction. It is thus used to describe an interaction characterised by high dentist and high patient control. A relationship characterised by mutuality results in both the patient and the professional regarded as experts. Such shared expertise is possible because the knowledge brought to the interaction by the patient interacts with the clinical skill and knowledge of the professional. This was certainly not the type of relationship which characterised the patient–dentist interaction in either of the cases discussed in this chapter.

Another of Stewart and Roter's types – the consumerist relationship – is not applicable to the cases described in this chapter. In each case, the women were seen by the clinical psychologist following their consultation with the dentist, – the referral was, however, instigated by the dentist. Neither of the women had exercised their prerogative as clients or as consumers. They had been directed to the clinical psychologist because their wishes were seen as inappropriate by the dentists involved. The women had not made requests for alternative opinions, as customers might if they felt unsure about the service they had received in the marketplace.

The final type of relationship, the default in Stewart and Roter's model, describes a situation where both the professional and the patient take little control in the interaction. The interaction is unbalanced because neither person in the interaction meets the other's expectations. As in the paternalistic and consumerist relationships, the imbalance of control usually results in an unsatisfactory outcome.

It is however important to be aware that not all patients wish for the degree of control these two women might appear to have wanted. Many patients are content with a paternalistic relationship. While a low degree of patient control might indeed meet these patients' expectations, the passivity which is associated with this model is not always desirable to the dentist. There must therefore be a variation in the degree of participation that is entered into by both parties.

The remainder of the chapter therefore considers clinicians' views on the characteristics desirable in patients.

Patients

A patient has been described as 'a kind of hearty hybrid who is three-quarters patient and one-quarter physician. They've learned to speak the doctor's [or dentist's – *authors' addition*] own language, and ask him questions rather than passively sit, honour and obey ... They've learned Body Talk – that special language of symptoms that enables them to know what an ache or pain is saying. And they are playing an important and needed role in health partnership with doctors [or dentists]' (Sehnert & Eisenberg 1975).

Such attitudes and behaviour on the part of patients, while welcome as an indication of motivated concern regarding their own health, would perhaps be regarded as a form of direct challenge to many professionals.

As the woman patient in the first case (3a) showed, asking questions of professionals can be fraught with difficulties, particularly if such questioning is seen as a challenge to what many regard as their traditional authority. However, as Armstrong (1984) stresses, by learning to accept what Balint (1964) termed 'the offers' which arise in discussion with the patient, the professional is actually seen by the patient as possessing more rather than less expertise.

The patient from the second case (3b) would certainly have found great difficulty in moving from what amounted to a default relationship with the dentist to one characterised by such a high degree of mutual participation (Sehnert & Eisenberg 1975). An alternative and perhaps less threatening view of patients is to describe them as 'active patients' who reject the sick role (which is passive), but assume responsibility for their care in the following way:

- Asking questions
- Seeking explanations
- Stating preferences
- Offering options
- Expecting to be heard.

All of these characteristics would provide a particularly well balanced and ideal patient!

Other characteristics that clinicians prefer to see in their patients include the following: similar or younger age to themselves, accepting of the diagnosis, compliant with instructions and able to pay fees for work completed. However, time and cost too often place constraints on the service dentists are able to offer their patients. The following chapter returns to the patient–dentist interaction. Attention is drawn to the system of providing dental care and how this can influence, sometimes adversely, the encouragement of a caring relationship between the clinician and patient. The physical environment acts as another constraint, including the reception and surgery areas. However, what is also important is recognising that the clinician not only gives information appropriately, but also empathises with the patient (i.e. recognises and expresses the emotional concerns of the patient).

References

Armstrong D 1984 The patient's view. Social Science and Medicine 18:737–744

Ayer W 1982 The dentist patient relationship. International Dental Journal 32:56–64

Balint M 1964 The doctor, his patient and the illness. London: Pitman Medical

Cohen A 1994 Self consciousness: an alternative anthropology of identity. London: Routledge

Cooley C 1902 Human nature and the social order. New York: Scribners

Croucher R 1989 The performance gap. London: Health Education Authority

Davis P 1976 Compliance structures and the delivery of health care: the case of dentistry. Social Science and Medicine 10:329–335

Eley B M 1998 The future of dental amalgam: a review of the literature. BDJ Books, London

Freidson E 1970 The profession of medicine: A study of the sociology of applied knowledge. New York: Harper Row

Green T, Lang W, Jacobson J 1988 Patient preference for forms of address. Journal of Dental Education 52:255–258

Grytten J, Rostow I, Steele L, Holst D 1988 Aspects of the formation of dental health behaviours in early childhood. Journal of the Institute of Health Education 26(2):62–68

Lahti S, Verkasalo M, Hausen H, Tuutti H 1996 Ideal role behaviours as seen by dentists and patients themselves and by their role partners: do they differ? Community Dentistry and Oral Epidemiology 24:245–248

Mead G 1934 Mind self and society. Chicago: University of Chicago Press

Parsons T 1951 The social system. New York: Free Press

Petersen P 1990 Social inequalities in dental health – towards a theoretical explanation. Community Dentistry and Oral Epidemiology 18:153–158

Reisine S 1981 Theoretical considerations in formulating sociodental indicators. Social Science and Medicine 15A:745–750

Sehnert K, Eisenberg H 1975 How to be your own doctor – sometimes. New York: Grossett & Dunlap

Stewart M, Roter D 1989 Communicating with medical patients. New York: Sage

Szasz T, Hollender M 1956 A contribution to the philosophy of medicine. AMA Archives of Internal Medicine 97:585–592

The dental team

The practice or clinic is the place where primary dental healthcare professionals spend most if not all their working day. Although trends in the delivery of oral healthcare are changing, so that domiciliary visits and clinics held in schools, offices and factories are not unusual, the majority of clinical interventions are conducted in the traditional setting where patients are invited to sit in the dental chair for examination and treatment. In order for clinicians to be able to work effectively, it is important to have some understanding not only of the clinical aspects of dentistry, but also of the social context and organisational framework within which dentistry is practised.

This chapter will therefore consider some features of the practice of dentistry within the British National Health Service (NHS), together with some of the different social processes and expectations which apply within primary dental care. The provision of dental care is increasingly being delivered by a range of dental staff that includes receptionist, hygienist, therapist, assistant and dentist. How these members can be integrated into providing a coherent service is discussed and an example provided of a team approach. The introduction of change and the increased demands on dental personnel may be a recipe for occupational stress.

Case 4a   The 'stressed' practice

A small internal study was conducted by a local dentist and his staff to assess stress and job satisfaction during the transition from the NHS system to an independent capitation scheme. All members of staff were encouraged by the principal to participate and this included the dentists, hygienist, reception and auxiliary staff. Initial results showed that the dentist had less job satisfaction than the other staff groups, which was a great surprise to the practice team. This result was explained by the dentist having to present the changes in the practice to the patients. Some concern was raised as a number of patients preferred to remain within the state system of care. Other interesting effects were those that served to increase pressures and were noticed by the team. For example, the practice was situated within a well defined urban area with a strong and close-knit community identity, and some members of staff were approached by local people in the shopping and recreational areas who expressed their dissatisfaction at the change in the 'neighbourhood' dental practice. These brief encounters were upsetting to staff resident in the area. Qualified dental staff were more able to argue the benefits of the changes and counter any negative responses. Less qualified staff with a stronger attachment in some respects to the local community found these interactions unpleasant and upsetting. The transition to the private insurance scheme was achieved within a year and the incidence of approaches from past patients to staff members stopped.

As case 4a demonstrates, general dental practice is changing and the process of change produces psychological effects on staff as well as patients. Such changes in the delivery of dental care can trigger wider social responses, which may also arise from public perception of a process of rapid change within the national provision of health care.

In order to understand these effects of changes in the delivery of dental care it is useful to appreciate some of the background to dental services in Britain. A brief overview is therefore provided of the development of dentistry within the NHS.

The dental service, established in 1948 with the introduction of the NHS, is provided predominantly within a primary care setting. NHS statistics for the 1990s indicate that around 80% of dentists work in the General Dental Service, around 10% practice in the Community Dental Service and a little less than 10% work within hospitals.

From 1948 until 1990, dentists working in the General Dental Service operated as independent practitioners paid from NHS funds on the basis of a fee-per-item of service provided to children and adults. Since 1951, some patients have had to pay a direct contribution towards the cost of their treatment. The range of patients having to contribute and the proportion of cost recouped from the patient has increased substantially in recent years. Currently, all approved dental treatment for children under 18 and for other selected groups with particular dental needs (such as pregnant women and nursing mothers) or with a low income (and in receipt of certain means-tested benefits) is provided free of charge.

The effect of dental charges on patients' willingness to seek treatment has been a matter of concern since their introduction in 1951. A report of the Guillebaud Committee in 1956 recognised that charges for dental treatment acted as a deterrent to some patients, although the Committee was unable to advise abolishing charges because of the financial implications for the NHS and the shortage of dentists at that time. Pressures on public finance have led to the continuation of charges and an unremitting trend of increases in the proportion of patients who are charged and of the cost recouped. By 1994 the proportion recouped had risen to 80% of the cost of each course of treatment up to a prescribed maximum charge of £275. The rising cost to patients of dental care has acted as one of the barriers to care (Finch 1988).

Although the General Dental Service originally provided care free at the point of delivery, and has remained free for some patients, it was never a universal service. It has only provided care for those people able to find a general dental practitioner who was prepared to treat them. The failure to provide guaranteed dental care for any individual arose because general dental practitioners operated as independent practitioners and were thus able to choose the location of their practice.

Some children and adults were therefore often subject to dental treatment that was episodic in nature. This arose because the dentist offering treatment to patients had no contractual responsibility to provide continuing care. The dentist's responsibility was rather to offer treatment which would ensure that patients were rendered dentally fit. Such an approach to care was very much focused upon a view of dentistry which emphasised repair and restoration rather than prevention of disease.

The new dental contract

In October 1990 a new dental contract (Department of Health 1990) for dentists working within the General Dental Services of the NHS resulted in changes to the basis upon which dentists were remunerated, and the introduction of a patient registration scheme. This scheme meant that patients who attended a dentist for more than just emergency treatment were able to enter into a longer term contractual relationship (firstly of 24 months and later of 15 months) with their dental practitioner. It was hoped that one effect of the new contract would be 'to improve the oral health of the nation by encouraging patients to visit their dentists regularly, and dentists to practise preventive care' (Department of Health 1994).

Part of the changes in remuneration included a capitation payment system for the treatment of children. The capitation system meant that, based upon the age of the child, for each child registered, dentists would receive a fee which was independent of the amount of treatment provided. It has been estimated (Bloomfield 1992) that these fees account for about 20% of the annual remuneration of a typical dental practitioner.

Partly because dentists were successful in registering patients, the changes in the remuneration system resulted in increasing expenditure by the NHS which led to a substantial budget overspend in 1992. In response, the Department of Health reduced the fees paid for NHS dental work by some 7% which led to dentists receiving rather less money for the work they undertook. There were also increasing limits on the type of dental treatment that would be approved within the NHS and restrictions on the use of certain more expensive materials and procedures.

These changes created an environment within which a growing number of dental practitioners decided to seek alternative bases for practising outside the NHS. Some practitioners increased the proportion of patients whom they treated privately and restricted the number of patients treated under the NHS. Other dental practices decided to transfer all their patients from NHS treatment to forms of care funded by private dental insurance schemes. Such changes often provoked expressions of concern from those patients who either feared exclusion or who felt they could not afford, or were not prepared to pay the costs of private dental insurance.

The dental practice involved in this case had decided to introduce treatment based upon private dental insurance and to phase out NHS dental care. These changes produced responses within the dental practice staff partly as a result of the general psychological effects of change, but also as a result of the responses to those changes by patients and others in the community.

A significant report known as the Nuffield Report was published in 1993 (Nuffield Foundation 1993). This was drawn up to make recommendations on the staffing required for modern-day dentistry. Two major areas were highlighted which have implications for all dental personnel. First, attention was drawn to how staff within the General Dental Service could be utilised to the best effect. It was pointed out that dentists who receive lengthy training should not be expected to carry out routine treatment which staff with less intensive training could competently complete. The challenge for practices would be to get the right combination of staff, known as skillmix. Staff who were previously known as dental hygienists or dental therapists would be known as clinical assistants and be able to conduct simple treatments such as certain types of filling. The implementation of this recommendation required legal and professional changes. The second area to be highlighted by the report was the encouragement of practices to work more as a team, rather than as a sole individual clinician with support staff such as a nurse and a receptionist. In this respect the team approach tends to be pointing towards dental surgeries adopting a general medical practice model. From a sociological perspective such a change in the professional structures of the dental personnel will bring about potential realignment in the power relationships between staff members. For instance the new organisations representing the clinical assistants are likely to request a greater say in practice running and management. Psychologically, the relationship between staff may be enhanced by concentrating on good communication skills (see Chapter 6).

Personal dental service

A new development for the NHS is the introduction of the Personal Dental Service. The current remuneration system for dentists has been seen to be too inflexible for certain areas of dental health need, as defined by the profession within the UK. In order that plans can be implemented to deliver services to meet these needs, bids have been invited by the NHS. Pilot schemes were tested in 1998. The aim of this service is to encourage the provision of specific services for local circumstances. Combinations of General, Community and Hospital Dental Services are allowed. An example of such a scheme includes the combined general and community dental services in a locality to provide an extraction service for children emphasising relative analgesia as opposed to general anaesthesia. The Personal Dental Service will be sensitive to local decisions made by commissioners and health service managers in the locality of the community being served. Health authorities have been given instructions by the Department of Health to seek opinion from local community groups and organisations. Examples within the dental field are difficult to find although the needs of special groups (such as elderly people) with strong local organisations such as social services can help to drive these new developments to tailor them for the clients concerned.

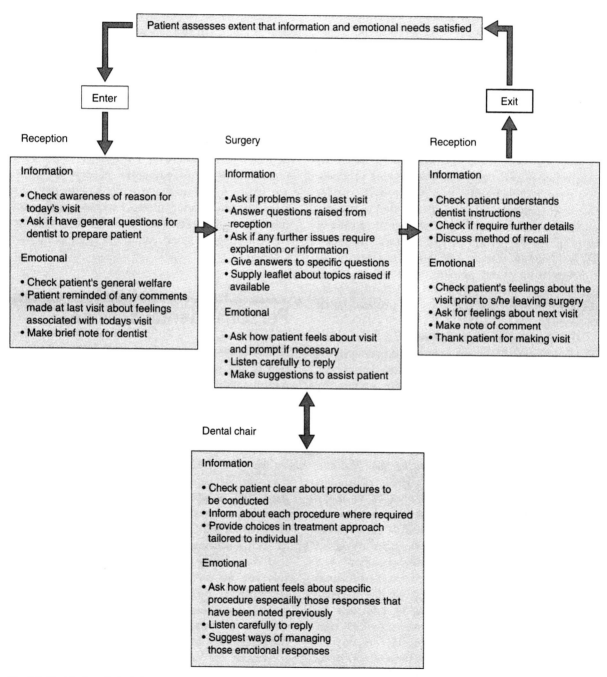

Fig 4.1 Model of psychological care.

PATIENTS NEED EMOTIONAL CARE AS WELL AS INFORMATION

The organisation of dental services to match local circumstances is a greater example of the pressures that exist at the clinic or practice level. When meeting patients face-to-face there are fewer barriers to communicating the sort of healthcare desired by the patient and what the dentist is prepared to offer. The case above (4a) indicates that some patients may exhibit quite strong psychological reactions to statements made by their clinician about treatment recommendations. Such reactions require sensitive communication skills in order to handle the depth of feeling with which some patients present. The success that the dentist and the practice staff make of appreciating the emotional content of the patient's difficulty or request will often determine the level of progress that is made in the treatment phase and ensures that the patient continues his attendance.

Fig 4.1 is a schematic diagram showing the types of task that a dental team might accept as a reasonable model of psychological care for patients. Such a model allocates tasks to three key areas of the practice or clinic, namely:

- The reception area
- The surgery
- The dental chair.

The tasks are divided into two categories referred to as:

- Information needs
- Emotional needs.

This follows the work of Nichols who stipulates that clinicians have to satisfy patients' desire for knowledge (about the condition of teeth and gums, treatments available and costs) as well as attending to their emotional concerns and responses (Nichols 1993). It is useful to separate these two aspects of patient:clinician interaction as different approaches are often required to provide for each category of need. The following example illustrates why this distinction is useful:

Dentist: I've completed your examination and as usual you have excellent oral hygiene, and the condition of your gums, as a consequence, is very good. However I have discovered from the radiograph, that is X-ray, I took earlier, that one of your back teeth requires a filling.

Patient: Oh dear, that's a pity – that will be the first filling I've needed to have. I'm proud of the fact that at the age of 32 my teeth have been perfect.

Dentist: Well there are different types of filling material that we can use, the traditional amalgam or the 'white' filling material. Sorry about this but I need to make a brief phone call in the next room. I will only be gone a few minutes. In the meantime perhaps I could ask you to look at a leaflet that my nurse has available for you to look at? You will find more details of these two types which will give you plenty of information.

A full explanation to a patient about the merits of different filling materials will probably not assist this patient. From the transcript it would appear that the patient is upset at the prospect of receiving a filling in the first place. It would be important to first identify the worry which the patient experiences by inviting him to express his fears of receiving a restoration.

The dentist could have responded in the following manner:

Dentist: I think you should be very proud of having been clear of dental decay, completely, well into your adult life. So I am sorry that I am having to give you some bad news about this tooth decay. What would you like me to do? I can show you the X-ray film if you like, which I hope will convince you that we should not leave it for too long before we treat it. I can also give you information on these various filling materials if you'd like? Shall I ask my hygienist to go over with you any questions you might have about preventing any future decay?

Note that the dentist has listened carefully to what the patient has said and picked up that the patient was upset about receiving a first filling. The dentist then gives an opportunity to the patient to respond to a series of questions. Alternatively the dentist could have paused after the question: 'What would you like me to do?' and given the patient wider scope to reply. The manner in which the dentist asked this question would be vital. For instance the question proposed, quietly and softly spoken would ensure a sensitive approach.

To summarise the model presented in Fig. 4.1:

1. The receptionist may encourage patients to think about questions that they would like to ask prior to entering the surgery. A note could be made of specific issues that the patient is concerned about and passed to the dentist or hygienist immediately before the patient enters

the surgery. At one practice, for example, patients who indicate they are nervous prompts the receptionist to place an orange sticker on the case sheet. Care should be taken, however, not to treat this system too literally as patients may legitimately regard such practice as stereotyping or labelling.

2. On entering the surgery the dentist or hygienist can make reference to the note or ask an open-ended question to start the patient session. Checking with patients if they have questions about a procedure or form of treatment and whether they have emotional concerns prior to examination or treatment will help a great deal in reducing dissatisfaction and conflict.

3. A system which collects patient concerns, or requests for information, at various stages during the dental visit, will send an important message to the patient that the dental personnel of the practice/clinic have attempted to deliver a high quality service.

4. Note that when the patient leaves the surgery, an assessment of needs being satisfied is conducted. Studies of satisfaction with services are popular. However, they produce data that very often report enthusiastic responses from the members of the public. Patients tend to generalise when asked non-specific questions about a service and appear to give the benefit of the doubt and a positive appraisal. It is better to ask patients what happened when they last went to the dentist and refer to specific events if at all possible. A wider range of answers is usually gained with this approach.

The previous chapter raised the issue of expectations of both the patient and the clinician and how conflicts arise in the interaction between the two individuals. Where the focus is centreed only on the patient, a complication arises in assessing patient satisfaction levels. How satisfied patients are will depend on their expectations. Patients with low service expectations may give a positive report to a visit which other patients with higher expectations would rate as unsatisfactory. The dental team member should however remember that patients have two major psychological needs, namely the need for appropriate information and for emotional care.

Analysis of dental visiting behaviour

It can be a heart-searching exercise for the person under training or newly trained to try and understand why patients fail to attend for an appointment. For instance you may be worried that you failed to put the patient at ease at his last appointment, or that you put him off in some way. Even experienced dental personnel are heard to say that they are bemused as to why a well-known patient suddenly decides to stop attending and switches practice. It is important that you remain sensitive to your concern for the patient. There may be ways that you can change your behaviour or that of the practice or clinic to encourage patients to visit and maintain their visiting in the future. To help you organise your thinking, try to adopt a broad screening of the factors that may be responsible – many are referred to in this book. The use of behaviour analysis is particularly helpful. This method can assist in drawing together the various factors that help describe whether a person will make a visit to the dentist. For instance, as shown in Fig. 4.2 not only does meeting requirements for information and emotional care following a dental visit define the consequences of that visit, a variety of other factors impinge on the individual which help set up conditions (i.e. antecedents) which may increase the likelihood of that visit being made.

A similar approach may be applied to other dental health behaviours (such as the use of floss or parental use of fluoride drops for children) and is especially useful when trying to understand and improve patient compliance (Weinstein et al. 1996). An example of using positive reinforcement in the dental field was reported in a study in rural North America. It adopted strict principles of behaviour analysis. It attempted to crudely alter families' decisions to make a visit to the local publicly-owned dental service for low income households (Reiss, Piotrowski & Bailey 1976). A number of families with young children were identified and randomised to three methods of encouragement to visit the service. The first was a simple letter of invitation which encouraged a minimal response (less than 20%). The second approach was to make

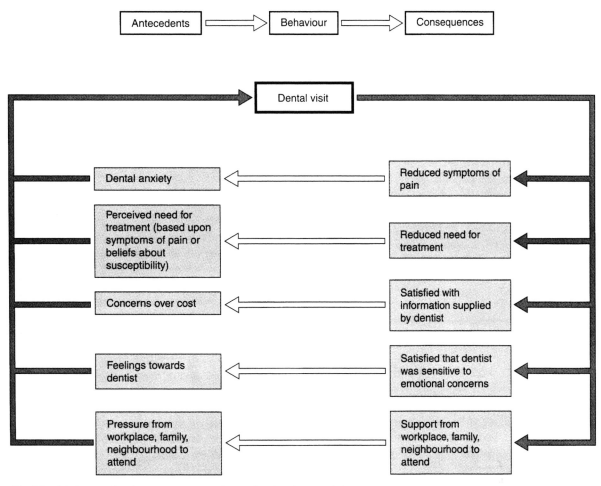

Fig 4.2 A behavioural-analytic approach to understanding dental visiting behaviour.

three prompts, including a letter of invitation, a telephone prompt and, following failure to attend, a visit to the home concerned to encourage an appointment to be made. The final approach was again a letter of invitation plus a monetary voucher ($5) redeemable on visiting the dental clinic. The three prompts and the monetary condition (i.e. second and third approaches) were found to encourage the same level of visiting (approximately 60%).

Interestingly the number of follow-up visits from the monetary voucher group far outweighed those from the other two groups, even though the voucher was a one-off experiment. A cost effectiveness analysis where a comparison of the costs between each of the approaches was made showed that the voucher scheme was a cheaper option per visit than the multiple prompt scheme (which was likely to encourage increased visiting by families feeling they were being victimised). Such approaches are not necessarily advocated as a more flexible supply of services may solve uptake problems, for instance the use of mobile surgeries, school inspections and workplace schemes.

This was a crude but important study. It was able to demonstrate the influence of positive reinforcement. Monetary reward is not a mechanism considered appropriate to encourage changes in health behaviour, for obvious fiscal reasons related to the public purse. However other reinforcers are available which include the use of praise by the dental team for the patient making the effort to visit the surgery. The creation of a pleasant and relaxed atmosphere within the practice or clinic is one example of a generalised reinforcer that would encourage reattendance. In addition the behaviour of the dental team as outlined in the 'information and emotional needs' model above would function as positive reinforcement for many who visited. A friendly confident manner exhibited by dental team members is likely to be reinforcing for many patients, but interestingly perhaps not all. All individuals have their own needs, wants and sensitivities. These can be expressed in terms of degrees of reinforcement. Some patients prefer a straightforward approach and suspect a lack of genuineness in staff who exhibit over-confidence. What is likely to give strong positive reinforcement to patients visiting the practice or clinic is a highly responsive staff who can be flexible to individual patient requests.

Stress in dentistry

The nature of the work in which dentists engage is subject to a variety of demands: from the dentist, the dental team, the patient and the wider community. Dentists and their team members may also experience strong psychological responses such as anxiety, anger, disappointment and frustration, in the course of their work. The previous case, for example, illustrates that some reactions to changes in the dental system of care produce adverse effects on staff. This area has come under increasing scrutiny.

Case 4b   The 'stressed' practitioner

A newly qualified dentist who had completed his initial vocational training was working full-time in a busy dental practice. During training, when he was under pressure, he experienced tension headaches. He had recently married and moved into a new house with the increased responsibility of paying a sizeable mortgage. He felt fairly fit but was not able to go to the local gym as often as he used to. His usual response to work pressure was to have a drink to relax. His employer was an experienced general dental practitioner who ran a mixed practice of NHS, insurance scheme and private patients. A hygienist and receptionist were employed. The young dentist experienced difficulties when the principal of the practice left the surgery at fairly short notice and expected his young colleague to take over. This resulted in the new recruit seeing a large number of patients he had to treat quickly, without supervision. The dilemmas facing him were not knowing when he would be asked to assume responsibility for the practice and a constant increase in workload. He felt pleased that such faith had been invested in him by his employer but the weight of responsibility was high. He had begun to experience a stiff neck, upper back pain and headaches. This worried him as there was a history of heart disease in his family.

Psychologists have identified many causes of stress that do not necessarily refer to the work situation. People vary enormously in response to stressors or pressures in their lives. It is true that there is an optimum level of demands placed upon people who work. A feeling of distress may be apparent in individuals where demands are either too low or high. Some of the causes are listed below and are apparent from the case above.

- Individual differences. We all have different susceptibilities to pressure and will respond more or less rapidly than others as shown by increases in heart rate, sudden perspiration, muscle tone and tension.
- When presented with an apparently insoluble problem this may, if we are not prepared, increase stress levels very highly. Examples include being given too little time to finish a task; being faced with a situation that has been set up to fail; being unable to predict an outcome; being presented with a task beyond your skill level, or beyond your control.
- Stress can be caused when there is too much change at once.
- A lack of feedback or emotional support and social reinforcement for actions will raise and maintain stress levels.

- Being forced to act in a way which is contrary to your key values, is a stress-heightening factor.
- A situation requiring constant awareness and concentration because there is a high risk of error (e.g. molar endodontics) provides the right conditions in the longer term for increasing stress.

For the health professional there are special features which may be regarded as additional pressures (Atkinson et al. 1991). These include:

1. The fact that health professionals provide a very individual service, meeting patients on a one-to-one basis.
2. Contact with people in distress and suffering from disease.
3. The health service is subject to change as a result of improved treatments and new management initiatives.
4. Challenges are being made to professionalism including to what extent specialists are needed in preference to generalists.

SPECIAL FEATURES OF DENTISTRY AND STRESS

According to a UK national study of general dental practitioners (Cooper, Watts & Kelly 1987) 'the stress levels in the profession are high, likely to go higher and are already having effects both in deteriorating levels of mental wellbeing and in the significant numbers of general dental practitioners with low levels of job satisfaction'. Cooper's research identified the medical emergency as the greatest source of stress for both male and female GDPs. Unco-operative patients, running behind schedule, constant time pressures, and dealing with very nervous patients were ranked highly by both sexes. Another interesting finding from this work was the extent to which the needs of the practice in terms of scheduling, income, staffing and quality control were prime concerns, with the potential for raising stress levels. These practice concerns tended to be more salient to dentists than concerns either for themselves or for patients. A study of general dental practitioners using in-depth interviews in the north-west of England in 1996, compared results with an original study ten years earlier, and found that some novel stressors could be identified (Humphris & Cooper 1998). These new pressures included coping with NHS system changes, higher patient expectations and hostile and aggressive behaviour towards staff in the practice.

An earlier study by American investigators demonstrated that 75% of a representative sample considered the practice of dentistry more stressful compared with other professions (O'Shea, Corah & Ayer 1984), and only 5% considered their work as less stressful. There is a strong general belief that dentists regard their potential for suicide to be greater compared with other professions (Kent 1987). However, the evidence for this belief is far from clear. In a careful review of the literature Kent quotes a number of surveys that have investigated the suicide rates of dentists across the Western world. The quality of the studies varies as they very often base their estimates of suicide risk on extended periods of time pooled together to provide sufficient data to calculate, confidently, rates of suicide. The problem is easily appreciated. For example, the extension of a five-year to a ten-year study period will make the suicide level calculated further removed from the present day. A calculation of suicide risk for British dentists found that the rate was lower than expected (Hill & Harvey 1972). Suicide levels are therefore not good indicators of stress within a profession, because the levels are so low that it is difficult to interpret these figures meaningfully. More work on occupational stress does however, need to be conducted. Demands on dentists may have increased in recent years, but so possibly has the recognition of stress and depression. In addition, the willingness of people generally to admit to experiencing signs of duress may have increased. Reasons for early retirement have been studied in 393 dentists in the UK as an exercise to identify whether stress-related illnesses were implicated (Burke Main & Freeman 1997). Anxiety and depression were responsible for 17% of early retirements which was the third most common cause after musculoskeletal disorders (30%) and cardiovascular disease (21%). There were some suggestions from the data at the time of major administrative change in the NHS dental system that the proportion of dentists retiring for nervous disorders was 25%.

BURNOUT

Occupational stress has been reported in many fields of work apart from dentistry, medicine and nursing. Studies of teachers, tax inspectors and air traffic controllers have shown that every job appears to have a stress 'footprint'. This can be translated as meaning that specific jobs have an identifiable set of stressors common to that job. Another way of examining a person's negative response to their work in the clinical field is to find out whether the person is suffering 'burnout'. This is a term employed to refer to those who work closely with patients, providing a caring service. It is believed that through the sheer number of patients, problems encountered and lack of support or value associated with the service, healthcare professionals become emotionally exhausted and 'hardened'. Cherniss (1982) has defined burnout as 'a process in which a previously committed professional disengages from his or her work in response to stress and strain experienced in the job'.

The definition given by Cherniss makes explicit that burnout is a process rather than an end state. Maslach takes this view further and regards burnout as a state that is composed of three elements (see Box 4.1). Each element is independently assessed: if all are present – namely depersonalisation, emotional exhaustion and personal non-achievement – this constitutes burnout (Maslach & Jackson 1986). The state of burnout is therefore dependent on personal contact in a service setting. Burnout can only occur in situations where members of the public make demands of the individual that require some emotional response and is therefore different to occupational stress which can apply to any job. A difficulty with the burnout construct is that one aspect may have rewarding consequences for the clinician – at least in the short term. For instance in junior hospital staff it appears that depersonalisation is adopted as a means of getting through a clinical rotation in the short term by distancing themselves from the concerns expressed by their patients. The

consequences for the patient are however unlikely to be positive.

BOX 4.1   COMPONENTS OF BURNOUT

Emotional exhaustion (EE) A strong sense of fatigue and lack of energy in associating with patient requests for emotional support or advice.

Depersonalisation (DP) Clinician exhibits a distancing from patient/client when interacting during an examination or treatment session.

Personal accomplishment (PA) Clinician has an overall feeling of achieving considerable goals in the job. This component will be negatively associated to the first two components: EE and DP.

Burnout Defined quantitatively by Maslach & Jackson as that state when the respondent has obtained scores on all three components above the upper tertial (i.e. above the level of the lower two-third of respondents).

A study of burnout in general dental practitioners (conducted in the south-east of England) has found that 11% experienced clearly defined levels of burnout as assessed by the Maslach Burnout Inventory (Osborne & Croucher 1994). Respondents to this self-report questionnaire had to record a certain profile of scores on three elements mentioned above: emotional exhaustion, depersonalisation and personal non-achievement. Burnout among junior hospital dentists was found to be at a very similar level (10%) in a sample drawn from the north-west of England (Humphris et al, 1997). Of interest in this study was the difference in depersonalisation between the main three dental specialties – oral surgery, restorative and orthodontics. The lowest level of depersonalisation was found among the orthodontists, and this specialty may have a greater level of control over the management of their clinics. The other specialties (surgery and restorative) cannot withdraw from certain of their treatments after they have started (e.g. surgical procedure for extracting a tooth). Orthodontists however have the capacity to make adjustments to their treatment within the session. If they find their schedule has been delayed they can provide a simple procedure and leave the more complex work to the next appointment. Hence they perceive greater flexibility in controlling the organisation of their work.

In a questionnaire study, community dentists and dental surgery assistants from north Wales said they were relatively dissatisfied with their jobs when compared with other comparable occupational groups. This low level of satisfaction could be explained to a significant degree by the reduction in autonomy over their work which they had experienced recently. The introduction of the health reforms current at the time of the study was suggested as an explanation for the decline in autonomy (Humphris & Peacock 1992).

Other recent studies in the UK have added further detail to the picture of stress in practice, and in the community dental and hospital services. A study by Blinkhorn – who used focus group methods to collect verbatim responses to his questions – demonstrated that there was a considerable number of stressors both for dentists and the DSAs. These stressors were often very different according to which group of staff they belonged (Blinkhorn 1992). There was however, an agreement that each group misunderstood the other to a considerable degree and wanted other staff members to appreciate problems from their position. Considerable benefits may be expected when dentists attend to staff management as an important skill for developing and improving communication and reducing conflict and misunderstanding.

A qualitative and quantitative research project (see Chapter 11 for a detailed discussion of these methods) was conducted to compare the stress experienced by dentists working under two different systems of remuneration (NHS and Denplan). Interestingly no differences were found between the stress levels of the two types of practice as measured by the questionnaire (using a quantitative approach). Both groups of dentists ($n = 28$) felt that patient management, time pressures and staff and practice management were sources of stress, though the independent schemes felt that they were under less time pressure and

had less paperwork. The methods used to cope were limited to exercise and 'switching off from dentistry'. Some dentists recorded that the transition to independent schemes was stressful (Newton & Gibbons 1996).

DENTAL STUDENT STRESSORS

Student stressors include the traditional problems expected in students such as academic concerns (unable to learn everything, preparing for exams) but also psychosocial dimensions (including conflicts with classmates, being treated as immature, dealing with authority, unsympathetic instructors). Other sets of stressors include time concerns, isolation and financial worries (Sachs, Zullo & Close 1981). The introduction of new teaching methods into dental curricula (for example, problem-based learning) and economic changes whereby students pay a proportion of their academic fees, often incurring debts, are just two additional pressures which may require monitoring in future investigations of stress in students. A greater proportion of women are entering the dental profession, and the Cooper national survey showed that qualified female dentists were less stressed than their male counterparts. Greater competition for key posts in the future may, however, be just one of the factors that could make a distinction between male and female stress levels insignificant. Prevention of overly stressful situations should be advocated. It is therefore important that some assistance service is made available to students. This may consist of some form of informational resource as well as professional counselling sessions. Such interventions require careful planning as the student body will quickly determine if the offered support is not properly organised. Issues of confidentiality, training, supervision and necessary expertise are all factors which require predetermined policies and service protocols. Further methods are explored in the section below.

ALLEVIATING WORK PRESSURES

The use of anxiety or stress management programmes in organisations is now commonplace. The fact that they continue to be provided on a routine basis in many companies and to public service employees suggests that the circumstances that produce excessive work stress are not diminishing. Alternatively, the mobility of the workforce is sufficient that the organised programmes appeal to a new audience because there are always new employees to attend. A sceptical view is that the employers need to demonstrate that they are trying to do something to alleviate their workforce's stress levels. Organising a stress management programme may seem unrealistic for the dental practice, however some guidelines are worth drawing up for yourself and others in your immediate workplace. These include:

- Physical strategies, such as relieving general tension by using relaxation techniques; improving diet and reducing alcohol intake; establishing better physical working habits such as posture and ergonomic seating positions.
- Behavioural approaches can be successful and include: anticipating problems, taking greater control through use of appropriate assertiveness skills, and relaxation sessions using one the many audio cassette tutors which are commercially available.
- Adoption of problem-solving methods (e.g. time management) and taking sufficient rest and recreation (referred to as 'time-out').
- Cognitive approaches, that is, thinking carefully about your own individual approach to work, may also reduce the effect of occupational stress. These approaches include examining irrational ideas about work (for example, 'I must *never* say no to a patient's treatment request, however unreasonable, and if I do I am a total failure'), trying not to anticipate the worst (catastrophising) and setting out a long-term plan of future work by prioritising essential and realistic achievements.
- The support of family and friends is important, as well as support from professional bodies such as the national and local dental associations.

References

Atkinson J M, Millar K, Kay E J, Blinkhorn A S 1991 Stress in dental practice. Dental Update 18:60–64

Blinkhorn A S 1992 Stress and the dental team: a qualitative investigation of the causes of stress in general dental practice. Dental Update 19:385–387

Bloomfield K 1992 Fundamental review of dental remuneration. Report of Sir Kenneth Bloomfield. Department of Health, London

Burke F, Main J, Freeman R 1997 The practice of dentistry: an assessment of reasons for premature retirement. British Dental Journal 182:250–254

Cherniss C 1982 Staff burnout, job stress in the human services. Beverley Hills: Sage

Cooper C L, Watts J, Kelly M 1987 Job satisfaction, mental health and job stressors among general dental practitioners in the UK. British Dental Journal 162:77–81

Department of Health 1990 The new dental contract. London: HMSO

Department of Health 1994 Improving NHS dentistry. London: HMSO

Finch E 1988 Barriers to the receipt of dental care. Social and Community Planning Research, London

Hill G B, Harvey W 1972 Mortality of dentists. British Dental Journal 132:179–182

Humphris G M, Cooper C 1998 New stressors in GDPs in the North West of England. British Dental Journal 185:404–406

Humphris G M, Lilley J, Broomfield D, Kaney S 1997 Burnout among junior staff of three dental hospital specialities. British Dental Journal 183:15–21

Humphris G M, Peacock L 1992 Occupational stress and job satisfaction in the community dental service of north Wales: a pilot study. Community Dental Health 10:73–82

Kent G 1987 Stress amongst dentists. In: Firth-Cozens J Payne R (eds.) Stress in health professionals. Chichester: John Wiley

Maslach C, Jackson S E 1986 Maslach burnout inventory. Palo Alto: Consulting Psychology Press

Newton J T, Gibbons D E 1996 Stress in dental practice: a qualitative comparison of dentists working within the NHS and those working within an independent capitation scheme. British Dental Journal 180:329–334

Nichols K A 1993 Psychological care in physical illness (2nd edn.) London:Chapman & Hall

O'Shea R M, Corah N L, Ayer W A 1984 Sources of dentists' stress. Journal of the American Dental Association 109:48–51

The Nuffield Foundation 1993 Education and Training of Personnel Auxiliary to Dentistry. The Nuffield Foundation

Osborne D, Croucher R 1994 Levels of burnout in general dental practitioners in the southeast of England. British Dental Journal 177:372–377

Reiss M, Piotrowski W, Bailey J 1976 Behavioural community psychology: encouraging low-income patients to seek dental care for their children. Journal of Applied Behavioural Analysis 9:387–397

Sachs R H, Zullo T G, Close J M 1981 Concerns of entering dental students. Journal of Dental Education 45:133–136

Weinstein R, Tosolin F, Ghilardi L, Zanardelli E 1996 Psychological intervention in patients with poor compliance. Journal of Clinical Periodontology 23:283–288

The social context of dental care for elderly people

Introduction

The increase in the proportion of elderly people within the Western population is a phenomenon of the twentieth century. In 1901 the proportion of adults aged 65 years or more was 6%. This will increase to 16% by the year 2001. Three million people, that is 1 in 20, are currently 75 years of age or over. The aged-dependency ratio is also increasing (i.e. the ratio of the number of non-working elderly to active working participants). This was 29 per 100 in the UK in 1985 and will be 38 per 100 by 2005.

In this chapter, there is no intention of treating elderly people as a group, isolated from the general population. Rather we intend that by giving attention to their particular dental health needs, we shall encourage practitioners to offer forms of care which permit many older people to discard 'the mask of old age' and emphasise their 'personal selves' (Hepworth & Featherstone 1989).

Utilisation of dental services by the elderly

The latest UK Adult Dental Survey in 1988 showed a marked depreciation in regular attendance by age group, so that by 75 years or more, 7% are attending the dentist regularly (Todd & Lader 1991). It should be noted however that 81% of this age band in the survey were edentulous. However, when looking at the attendance rates over the last 20 years there appears to be a definite increase in the proportion attending regularly. National surveys show self-reported dental attendance for dentate adults only. It is difficult to assess attendance of edentulous people. Edentulousness increases with age. Fifty-seven per cent of those aged 65–74 years in the national survey referred to were without teeth in comparison with the 81% of those aged 75 years and higher. It is clear that edentulous people would benefit from occasional visiting to check the fit and state of their dentures and to screen for oral pathology. A recent study in Liverpool has reported that dentate people were six times more likely to perceive the need for treatment in comparison with edentulous individuals. Hence there is difficulty in determining how to encourage regular attendance patterns in edentulous people (Tickle & Worthington 1997).

ATTITUDES OF OLDER ADULTS

There is little agreement on what could be considered to be the general attitude towards dental health and dentistry among elderly people. However, with the increase of this population it would seem important to consider their views more carefully. The planning of dental services in the future will become more attuned to satisfying the demands of elderly people as levels of increased retention of natural teeth extend into people's more advanced years. In a large study of dentate adults ($n = 1211$) aged 60 years and above from three English communities it was found that men were less concerned about the prospect of being edentulous than women (Steele et al. 1996). Women were more likely to opt for restoration and make a visit to the dentist.

Of particular interest was the view expressed by the sample regarding the preservation of their remaining natural teeth. Overall the authors believed that their respondents had high expectations which may have implications for dentists in trying to meet these demands. Two attitudes, which appear to vary with age, may be seen with regard to using the dentist.

Firstly, the 'old-old' (i.e. 75+ years) tend to be less fearful of dentists but aspects of the dentist's image become a barrier. Concerns were also expressed by this group of people about whether 'fancy treatments' would be offered. Some patients also reported their dislike of lying flat in the chair (Todd & Lader 1991).

Secondly, a problem for many of this group of elderly people is maintaining contact with their dentist. A dentist's retirement or death may make finding a new dentist whom they can trust a likely problem.

Understanding older adults' beliefs about the need for treatment shows these beliefs to be dependent on recent symptomology (recent pain experience) and concern (an anxiety-related factor) about oral health and appearance.

ATTITUDES TO LOSING TEETH AND WEARING A DENTURE

For patients who have retained their natural dentition into their later years the prospect of losing teeth can be a great shock. It may remind them that in fact they are getting old and force them to face and unwelcome 'reality'. Breaking bad news is something all dentists are involved in at some time or other. The guidelines set out below apply equally to giving news about the loss of a tooth as to a potential malignant lesion of the oral mucosa. Fig. 5.1 lists points which are helpful in giving bad news making the mnemonic CLAIRA, (adapted from Lloyd & Bor 1996). The important skills to remember when breaking bad news is to check with the patient what they know already. It is also essential to find out how much the patient would like to be told, as people vary in the amount of information they wish to obtain. However, be prepared to give substantial levels of information as on the whole people prefer to have information, even when it can be distressing. Check to determine

the personal strengths of the individual to whom you are giving bad news. A patient who is extremely nervous or frail would not be in a good position to receive potentially upsetting information. It is important though not to use this as an excuse for delaying unnecessarily giving news to the patient. For instance, the practitioner may invite the patient to return and ask him to bring a friend or relative to discuss the issue. While giving the factual information, check with the patient that he understands what is being said and tackle his questions in a sympathetic manner. Do not crush all hope. Invite the patient to come again and inform others – for example colleagues in the practice – of the situation. Linked closely to the prospect of losing teeth is the distress felt by many elderly people that they will have to wear a denture. Surprisingly, those aged 65 years or more are the most upset at this (Todd & Lader 1991) possibly because they have managed to retain their teeth for so long and are losing them when they are least able to adapt. The following case illustrates some of the difficulties many people in such a position face.

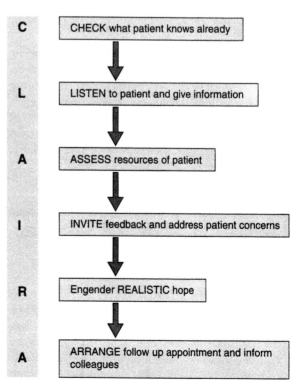

Fig 5.1 The breaking of bad news (adapted from Lloyd & Bor 1996).

Case 5a   Habit or chronological age?

This patient is 75 years old, and he has been attending the dental practice over a period of several weeks. He recently had all his permanent teeth extracted and was, as he described: 'trying to get the fine tuning of my new dentures right'. When he entered the dental surgery, he was accompanied by his wife. He was upset, and explained that his wife had accompanied him because 'Look, her dentures are a smashing fit! They're not like mine, all loose and wobbly.' He then demonstrated how his were 'loose and wobbly'.

The dentist asked the husband and wife to sit down. He brought an extra chair into the surgery and began to talk to the couple.

He was told by the woman that: 'He's only making a fuss. You see, he's not like me, I've had dentures since my early 40s, and I'm 75 now, like my husband, but I've got used to them.'

The dentist explained to the patient that what his wife had said was certainly important. Many patients do find difficulty in getting used to dentures. However, he could understand how much more difficult it must seem to him because dentures were something new to cope with.

The patient then assumed that the dentist was attributing his difficulties to his age. It was age that was making adapting to the new situation difficult. However he went on:

'I suppose things like this can happen when you're my age. But I don't really see why it should. After all I may have lived for 75 years or more, but I don't feel any different. I still play golf three times a week, drive my car and go abroad on holiday, so why should teeth cause me all this bother?'

The dentist was then able to reassure this patient that his age was not the central issue, rather it was habit, i.e. the length of time he had been used to having his own teeth. Like anything else he was unfamiliar with, there was a likelihood that it would cause him

some difficulty or concern. Indeed his wife was able to remind him of the problems she had had, getting used to her new dentures 30 years ago. She too had spent some time despairing about the loss of her own teeth.

The patient then agreed that he was prepared to have some adjustments made to his dentures. He returned a few weeks later for a final appointment. He thanked the dentist for his attention, making a final comment: 'Yes they do fit a lot better, and I am getting used to them, but I don't care what anyone says, your own teeth are the best.'

There are other factors which may be important in determining attitudes towards loss of teeth and the functional limitations that will result. In a recent study of older adults from two Liverpool electoral wards – one being the most deprived in the city and the other the most affluent – it was found that the level of impairment (per cent edentulous) was higher in the deprived ward compared with the affluent ward. However the psychosocial impact (that is, the ability to chew, speak clearly, suffer pain and other oral symptoms) was very similar across the two localities which was contrary to expectations (Tickle, Craven & Worthington 1997). The work of sociologist David Locker in Canada suggested that deprived areas would show significant self-reported functional and psychosocial problems as a result of a high level of dental impairments. The Liverpool study was however surprising. It indicated few differences and presented evidence to show that functional problems such as pain and chewing ability were more closely related to the psychosocial impact of impairment than socio-demographic variables such as education and those which indicate deprivation, for example unemployment, over-crowding, low levels of car ownership, etc.

The authors explain the lack of difference in psychosocial effects of dental impairment between the two electoral wards by saying that the origins of psychosocial problems may be different between the two areas. The deprived ward may consist of people who suffer high levels of general psychological distress and do not attend closely to the poor condition of their oral health, whereas the more affluent dental patient, who wishes to keep his teeth, is more concerned about the possibility of a dental health problem and becomes upset at the prospect of his dental health being compromised.

In the only longitudinal study to date on older adult perceptions of oral health it was interesting to find that the older person's view of their oral health was unrelated to clinical oral health status (Locker 1997). The only exception to this was tooth loss. It was predicted that the loss of a tooth would nearly always be regarded as a negative event. Those who had lost a tooth (as opposed to not losing a tooth) were more likely however to view their mouths as *either* worse or better off. This finding also tends to go against expectations. A deterioration or improvement in self-perceived health with tooth loss is difficult to explain. However, the condition of the lost tooth was not recorded, therefore the individual whose tooth may have been causing symptoms such as pain would welcome the removal of the tooth. The person with a tooth that was asymptomatic but was unsaveable due to its poor periodontal condition would cause him or her to become upset. This might explain such a finding.

COMPARING 'NEW' VS. 'OLD' ELDERLY

The expectations of elderly people are changing with respect to retention of natural teeth. Even in the last ten years (Todd & Lader 1991) dramatic increases in expectations from 1978 to 1988 have been demonstrated in the 65+ years population, especially among people with only natural teeth (that is, 68% in 1978 compared with 82% in 1988 expect to retain their natural teeth for life). The 'new' elderly have experienced more up-to-date dentistry, aimed at restoring rather than removing teeth and are therefore demanding more positive dental treatment (Ettinger & Beck 1982).

BARRIERS TO DENTAL CARE FOR ELDERLY PEOPLE

As among the general population, there are several difficulties faced by elderly people who require dental care. One important set of barriers exists with regard to participating in treatment – this set of barriers involves issues about access and mobility as well as perceptions of treatment need. The other set of barriers is concerned with age-linked expectations.

Treatment barriers

Among elderly people above the age of 75+ years and living independently there are a substantial number of barriers to utilisation (MacEntee-Dowell & Scully 1988). Unlike the patient in Case 5a, the majority of a large UK sample of 75-year-old people (54%) were found to have a chronic health problem. Sixty-nine per cent used prescribed medication daily. A third said they would need help to get to their dentist. Nearly half reported an oral health complaint, and nearly a third experienced pain. However, 57% had not been to the dentist for ten years, and had not been because they felt there was 'nothing wrong'. Two per cent only had been visited by their dentist at home, while 22% would have liked a dentist to visit them. Hence poor mobility and a lack of concern for teeth appear to be major barriers. Similar conclusions can be drawn from a study in Halton Health Authority (Hoad-Reddick, Grant & Griffiths 1987) who reported from a survey of elderly people resident in different types of accommodation. If resident in a long-stay hospital a small percentage only (44%) were aware of their local dentist. Mobility problems were also cited. The majority rated a dental visit as unnecessary. This was also borne out in the study by Steele and co-workers already mentioned: these authors found that the strongest reason for not attending a dentist was the perception of lack of need (Steele et al. 1996).

Another very important barrier for elderly people is that created by stereotypical thinking about old age. The patient in Case 5a conveyed an awareness of such stereotypes.

Ageist stereotypes

Ageist stereotypes reveal an insensitive, rigid or inflexible way of thinking about older people that results in discriminatory attitudes and assumptions about their capabilities. Sometimes an assumption is made that older people are no longer active participants in the community. They are seen as confined to a group or subculture because they hold their own norms and values which may be different from those held by the majority of society. However, elderly people are not uniform in terms of lifestyle. As with any other segment of the population they may vary according to class, gender or ethnicity.

Withdrawing or disengaging from society was the basis of an important theory put forward to explain how people age (Cumming & Henry 1961). This theory suggests that ageing has certain fixed physical, psychological and social effects, although as the following examples show, it is flawed.

Physical impairments

Elderly people are more subject to chronic diseases which may have an important bearing upon maintenance of oral hygiene or denture care. Stroke damage may prevent fine motor movements of the arm and hand to use oral hygiene aids (see Case 5b). However, it is important not to attribute certain oral changes to old age: reduced salivary flow, changes in oral mucosa and musculature are not likely to be a result of old age but an active pathological process which warrants investigation.

Psychological impairments

Depression is common among elderly people. Lack of motivation and lethargy are features which will compromise oral health through lack of oral hygiene, though strategies can be adopted to improve such situations. Dementia may influence treatment planning at the mid to later stages of this degenerative disease, but detailed assessments can be undertaken to determine the level of intervention when treatment is indicated. Support for the carer by providing information is especially helpful. Visits to homebound or institutionalised patients are greatly appreciated by carers and residential staff where mobility is compromised. Effective collaboration with other health professionals is also extremely important, particularly because of the multifaceted nature of such illnesses.

How these different types of impairment operate in practice – and some of the resolutions

that are available – are evident in the case of an elderly male patient who had suffered a stroke.

Case 5b   Management of oral hygiene in a stroke rehabilitation patient

A psychogeriatrician was concerned about the management of a 75-year-old man (Mr Stainer) who had suffered a severe stroke and was being cared for at home by his long-suffering wife. At a home visit the clinical psychologist interviewed Mrs Stainer and met Mr Stainer. He was unable to speak, though he attempted to shake hands in greeting. Mrs Stainer had been looking after him for over a year but was having difficulty with washing, shaving and brushing his teeth. He was just able to walk with assistance around the ground floor of their home (his bed had been moved downstairs to the front room). His wife's main difficulty was his disruptive behaviour in the bathroom. On occasion he would shout and push his wife away. This behaviour she found most upsetting as she felt his grooming was an important part of his retaining his identity and self-respect. On questioning it was apparent that this disruptive behaviour was most likely during his toothbrushing routine. Mrs Stainer described that she had to brush his teeth for him as she believed him to be incapable. She agreed to keep a brief diary of her husband's behaviour over a three-week period (19 days were recorded). The first week was regarded as a baseline. Two changes were suggested to Mrs Stainer to assist in the management of her husband's behaviour. She was asked what activities she believed her husband still enjoyed, and she replied that he smiled and attempted to sing to music. It was recommended that she bring the tape-cassette player into the bathroom and play a favourite piece of his music. She was also advised to encourage her husband to brush his own teeth. Although his ability to brush may not be fully effective it was explained to Mrs Stainer that her insistence on performing his toothbrushing herself may be precipitating his aggressive reactions.

From observation of the diary records presented in diagrammatic form (see Fig. 5.2) the intervention appeared to have an effect on reducing Mr Stainer's disruptive behaviour. For example the average number of disruptive behaviours per day in the first week was 2.9, whereas for the intervention period of 12 days the average was 1.2. From 'eyeballing' the diary record it can be seen that the degree of disruption of the toothbrushing routine was not great before the intervention. On interviewing Mrs Stainer the impression had been gained that the problem was more frequent. However no instance occurred following the change of management. An alternative explanation may be offered: the toothbrush clamping may already have reduced to near zero level before formal recording. The other behaviours were more frequent at baseline and did not extinguish entirely during the intervention period. Some evidence is indicated that the husband vocalised more at the start of the intervention and became more likely to fidget and push Mrs Stainer when being shaved. Record-keeping of this nature and attempting to interpret change is an example of 'behavioural analysis' which can assist in cases where there are strong emotional issues (for example his wife stated 'his disruptiveness shows he does not love me any more' and 'he just doesn't appreciate what I am trying to do for him').

There may be some truth in Mrs Stainer's statements but they would be very difficult to prove and painful for her to contemplate. A simpler explanation may be derived from careful observation that indicates a new plan of action to assist in changing behaviour. It is not clear in this case, of course, what element of this simple intervention was responsible for the modification in the husband's behaviour. Further diary-keeping would be preferable to ensure confirmation and maintenance of his behaviour change. The community dental service was informed to continue supporting this couple. It is important to note that the husband was included in discussions of the changes that his wife was going to introduce into his grooming routine. His difficulties in communicating however hindered his involvement in the design of the intervention. It is important to encourage input from the various parties involved to provide the best chance of implementation and positive results.

PSYCHOLOGICAL MANAGEMENT CONSIDERATIONS

Communication with elderly people may be difficult due to progressive loss of function of the brain, chronic depression, reluctance to talk to strangers or distrust of younger people. Continuity of care is to be stressed with disabled elderly patients where the dentist can have an important role in the overall wellbeing of the patient. Quality of life considerations should be attended to. Life expectancy, future medical status and the physical resources of the patient therefore need to be estimated. The aim should be to remedy adverse pathology and treat conditions which are handicapping patients in their daily life. The clinician should exercise 'rational' dental care, and take account of the attitudes of the patient's carer, and his or her willingness to assist in oral hygiene maintenance.

The dental care of the patient with Alzheimer's disease requires special consideration. Alzheimer's is an organic degeneration of brain tissue responsible for progressive dysfunctional loss of memory and thinking and eventually central functions such as walking, eating and continence. For carers the initial and middle phases produce the greatest burden. The initial phase, where the patient is aware of a gradual diminution of memory (especially short term) and lack of orientation of time and space, can produce crushing bouts of depression and apathy to self-care. The middle phase, where patients have less insight into their loss of cognitive abilities, show more dramatic limitations including an inability to recognise familiar objects and people (for example close relatives), loss of speech, increased wandering,

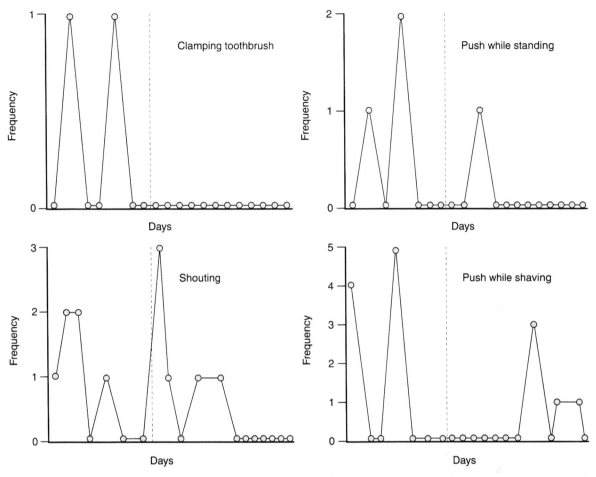

Fig.5.2 A diary of the frequency of four disruptive behaviours kept by the carer of a stroke patient. Assessment was conducted in the first 7 days (i.e. baseline period indicated by the points (prior to the vertical line) and for the next 12 days following the introduction of the intervention (after the vertical line), which was playing the patient's favourite music while allowing him to brush his teeth with minimal assistance from his carer.

disruptive behaviour and stereotypical behaviour patterns. The lack of awareness of objects and time can place severe strain on the carer who may have to cope with resistance from the patient to maintain a daily routine. The final phase is characterised by a severe reduction in all cognitive functions and extreme apathy. The patient will be confined to bed and be cared for in a more intensive serviced facility than could be provided at home. The patient will be easier to manage from a behavioural viewpoint because he will be subdued for a majority of the time. The dentist will need to institute a treatment plan that aims to restore oral function without delay for the initial visits of a patient in the first phase of Alzheimer's disease, and also adopt strong preventive measures such as

topical fluoride applications, frequent oral hygiene practices and education to caregivers (Niessen et al. 1985). These authors present a useful dental care index for the management of the patient with Alzheimer's disease.

ELDER ABUSE

An increasingly recognised and disturbing phenomenona now being met by healthcare workers is elderly people who show evidence of having been abused. Definitions vary about what constitutes elder abuse, some consensus is however being achieved and this includes both physical harm (bruising, fractures, burns) and psychological elements (name-calling, aggressive remarks, threats). Instances of neglect, fraud and unwanted sexual contact are often included in the institutional policies of watchdog agencies such as social services. The incidence of elder abuse has been estimated at about 3% although accurate levels are difficult to obtain due to the sensitive nature of the enquiry. However a report has shown that relatives who do abuse are often willing to admit their behaviour and request help (Homer & Gilleard 1990). This is most likely to be true of course if no legal implications are introduced. The victim of the abuse is unlikely to admit to there being a problem and in some cases will prefer if asked to remain in the environment even though still at risk of being abused. The abused elder person may often feel a greater fear of the solution offered by the care agencies than of continued victimisation by the abuser. An important point for dentists to be aware of is the possibility that they may be the first to spot evidence of abuse. Typical presentations will be various aspects of trauma: a dislocated or fractured jaw, traumatised or missing teeth or bruising, lacerations, ulceration or grazing from the brutal placing or removal of dentures. Neglect of dentition is probably not regarded as evidence of abuse but could be responsible for severe discomfort of the patient (pain from abscess, ill-fitting or missing denture). As found in the area of child abuse the cause of elder abuse is rarely attributable to the victim being difficult to care for. On investigation, the carer often has a catalogue of difficulties (alcohol abuse, drug use, previous evidence of violent behaviour). Those who work in the maxillofacial field should regard elder abuse as an area of concern with elderly patients who have sustained maxillofacial injuries due to a fall (Chew & Edmonson 1996).

Conclusion

People on average live longer than they used to. Older people therefore now comprise a large proportion of the population. Such change occurs because of advances in maintaining the human body in working order, and because of social influences. In order to provide effective dental treatment and services for this section of the population it is important that practitioners are aware of the dangers of ageist stereotypes. This enables treatment, which is based upon a patient's individual needs, to be offered and so to ensure that people remain full and active members of society for as long as possible.

References

Chew D W, Edmondson H D 1996 A study of maxillofacial injuries in the elderly resulting from falls. Journal of Oral Rehabilitation 23(7):505–509

Cumming E, Henry W 1961 Growing old. New York: Basic Books

Ettinger R, Beck J 1982 The new elderly: what can the dental profession expect? Geriatric Dentistry 2:62–69

Hepworth M, Featherstone M 1989 Ageing and old age. In B. Bytheway (ed.) Becoming and being old. London: Sage

Hoad-Reddick G, Grant A A, Griffiths C S 1987 Knowledge of dental services provided: investigations in an elderly population. Community Dentistry and Oral Epidemiology 15:137–140

Homer A C, Gilleard C 1990 Abuse of elderly people by their carers. British Medical Journal 301:1359–1362

Lloyd M, Bor R 1996 Communication skills for medicine. Edinburgh: Churchill Livingstone.

Locker D 1997 Clinical correlates of changes in self-perceived oral health in older adults. Community Dentistry and Oral Epidemiology 25:199–203

MacEntee-Dowell T, Scully C 1988 Oral health concerns in England. Community Dentistry and Oral Epidemiology 16:72–74

Niessen L C, Jones J A, Zocchi M, Gurian B 1985 Dental care for the patient with Alzheimer's disease. Journal of the American Dental Association 110:207–209

Steele J G, Walls A W G, Ayatollahi S M T, Murray J J 1996 Dental attitudes and behaviour among a sample of dentate older adults from three English communities. British Dental Journal 180(4):131–136

Tickle M, Craven R, Worthington H 1997 A comparison of the subjective oral health status of older adults from deprived and affluent communities. Community Dentistry and Oral Epidemiology 25:217–222

Tickle M, Worthington H V 1997 Factors influencing treatment need and the dental attendance patterns of older adults. British Dental Journal 182(3):96–100

Todd J E, Lader D 1991 Adult dental health: 1988 United Kingdom, OPCS Survey Division. London HMSO

PART 2

Enabling contact between patient and dental staff

6

Using communication skills

The ability to introduce yourself, listen to patient concerns and problems, explain procedures and treatments or ways of promoting health will be crucial to successful oral care. Traditionally these skills have been learnt by observing senior staff. Unfortunately the evidence for this 'osmosis' is scanty and with complaints against health personnel increasing it is recognised that some formal teaching in communication is necessary. Consequently many dental schools now have courses that teach clinical communication skills. These courses may vary considerably in where they appear in the curriculum, but they are often taught in small groups of students led by a tutor. Scenarios of common clinical situations with patients are rehearsed and practised using 'role play' (see Box 6.1). Trying new ways of solving problems in front of colleagues is not always easy; however, the advantage of sharing difficulties and of learning from each other is worth the initial reticence which may be felt by participants about this learning approach. The difficulties in clinical situations that are commonly raised by students in teaching sessions may be summarised below:

- Very talkative patients–or those who remain almost totally silent.
- Patients who become over-familiar or dependent.
- Patients who have very fixed opinions or beliefs about their dental health which is at odds with clinical examination and knowledge (for example, a request for all amalgam fillings to be replaced because of fear of mercury poisoning).
- Patients who become tearful (perhaps because of a recent bereavement in the family), distressed or anxious.

- Patients who do not follow advice such as oral hygiene instruction.
- Patients who make complaints: for example if they had to wait too long for treatment to be completed.
- Patients who are inconsistent in giving their past dental/medical history (for example, a partial history given when seen first by student, and a fuller history provided to a senior member of staff).
- Patients who need to be told something unpleasant or negative (such as giving the patient the news that their tooth cannot be saved, even after extensive attempts to restore it).

This chapter will assist you in your management of patients generally and encourage you to think about your own approach to them. Some of the difficulties mentioned above are not soluble simply with the use of appropriate communication skills. However, by becoming more aware of the part that communication skills can play in the dental consultation, the difficulties with patients presented above may be averted, or at least minimised.

BOX 6.1 ROLE PLAY

This is a procedure that is often used in communication skills teaching (CST). If you undertake a course of CST it is very likely that you will be invited to participate in role play exercises. A role play is a scenario in which there is usually a patient and clinician. The scenario is agreed before the exercise begins; they are either supplied by the teacher (sometimes known as the facilitator) or

---

offered by yourself, the student. Students can play the patient or clinician. Students who play the patient gain an advantage of what it feels like to be communicated to in the manner adopted by the clinician. The student who plays the clinician can experiment with various techniques or strategies in comparative safety, knowing that a real patient will not be upset. Safeguards will be put in place when you are involved in role play activity. For example, explicit rules of giving feedback to each other will be strongly adhered to in order to prevent damaging criticism. In addition, if students get 'stuck' in a role play, i.e. unsure what to say or do next, then he is advised to push an imaginary 'pause' button to seek advice from his peers. The method has great flexibility and immediacy. Some students find role play difficult as it appears artificial. This can be overcome by greater attention to providing more background detail about the scenario and making the objectives of the exercise clear before starting. Some role plays will include simulated patients. The use of simulated patients can be standardised for assessment purposes. Alternatively, specific difficult tasks can be assigned to students to practise in role plays, such as the giving of bad news.

What are communication skills and which are suitable for the dental context?

A good working definition of communication is offered by Brooks and Heath (1985) who state it is 'the process by which information, meanings and feelings are shared by persons throughout the exchange of verbal and non-verbal messages'. What specific skills should you possess to assist yourself and your patients in the delivery of good healthcare? Asking patients what they would like from their dentist is a good starting point. As has been outlined in Chapter 3, two of the ideal qualities that patients wish for in their dentist are

warmth and friendliness. Other sources indicate that to improve patient satisfaction and reduce dental anxiety (a major difficulty for many dental patients – see Chapter 7) patients put forward a number of suggestions, the majority of which are related to methods of communication. Patients' suggestions of things a dentist can do to reduce dental anxiety (Corah et al. 1988) are listed below:

- Prevent pain
- Show friendliness
- Working quickly
- Have a calm manner
- Give moral support
- Reassure about pain.

There is an overlap between communication skills and clinical skills. For example, patients request their dentist to work quickly. This preference appears to be against the general view of other clinicians (say medics) where patients on the whole complain of too little time being spent in a consultation. For these anxious patients, it is suggestive of an avoidance strategy being employed by the patient to reduce the experience of sitting in the dental chair. Evidence from surveys suggests that patients, regardless of being dentally anxious or not, like greater time in discussion with the dentist about their dental health, and seek reassurance about the treatment procedures they require.

Another approach to determining the communication skills required of all clinicians, and not only dentists, can be found from patient complaints. An early report from the NHS Ombudsman (1978) found virtual agreement in the 120 complaints they received. There were four problem areas:

1. Many health professionals restrict their information gathering to a very narrow set of concerns. Patients often feel that they are unable to express the problem they are really anxious about.
2. The information that is given to patients is often woefully inadequate. Clinicians may assume that patients know a great deal about their bodies and how they work, but unfortunately the evidence suggests otherwise. When patients are asked to indicate where fundamental organs are placed within the body

the percentage of correct answers received is low (Boyle 1970). Clinicians need to give more attention to ensuring that patients are informed *to the level they wish.*

3. Clinicians are not always good at 'sitting back' and listening carefully to their patients. It is this process which is so often neglected and can provide dramatic results in terms of improved diagnosis and increased levels of patient satisfaction.

4. The emotional concerns of patients are rarely elicited by the clinician. These concerns can often be managed relatively quickly and simply: by correction if the patient is misinformed, or at least by recognising with the patient the legitimacy of their worries so that the patient feels that at least he has been heard. The process of support provided by the clinician can provide a high level of assistance in helping the patient to cope with their symptoms, or difficulties in adhering to a programme of self-care or medication prescribed by the dentist.

More recently the Audit Commission report on Communication in Hospitals (1993) also presents a far from encouraging picture. The rudimentary communication skills employed by consultants observed in this investigation were patchy and in some cases non-existent. Instances where there are clear issues of communication skills for dental staff to be aware of include:

- Presenting oral hygiene instruction and dietary change.
- Providing explanations to assist certain forms of treatment for example, advice on stopping smoking to allow surgical procedures for periodontal disease or the provision of implants.
- Giving bad news (e.g. presenting to patients that teeth have to be removed when they are keen to retain their natural dentition).
- Negotiating with a parent and child over treatment procedures (for instance, encouraging the child patient to accept relative analgesia as opposed to general anaesthesia for the extraction of a tooth, say for orthodontic purposes).

Benefits of communication skills

Case 6a A positive patient story

Gender: Male   Age: 35   Occupation: Salesman

Problem: Toothache

Features: Patient has had four extractions over past two years

Attending the dental hospital for specialist investigation, this patient reported a recent visit to his new dentist:

My new dentist spent most of her time just listening to me for the first appointment and then decided not to take any teeth out. She also took some X-rays of my teeth. I was surprised as all of my previous dentists asked me a few standard questions, you know, age, previous treatment I'd had, how bad the pain was and how long I had experienced the pain. This dentist I go to see now is quite different. She asked me what I thought the pain was, what I wanted her to do, what effects previous extractions had had on the pain. I said that the pain tended to go down for a few days and then just come back as bad if not worse. What I liked about her was that she wanted to know my ideas and it made me feel very good that I had been listened to. I felt more inclined to tell her about the lousy time I was having at home and the worries about my wife's health and whether she was going to become housebound from her asthma attacks. I found myself not able to get the idea out of my mind that really the pain was a signal that something bad was festering away in my mouth. She very gently suggested that instead of taking any more teeth out she would ask me to go and see a specialist for further investigations. On thinking about it now she was very persuasive without having done a great deal. I just felt supported, in making the decision, to do as she suggested.

The benefits of clinicians adopting good communication skills are considerable. They are illustrated in the patient example above. The advantages are well documented and summarised in Box 6.2. The dentist that encourages the patient to describe explicitly his symptoms of discomfort from an aching tooth (for instance) will be in a better position to make a correct diagnosis. To invite the patient to give his opinion of what may be responsible for the pain will ensure that the dentist can correct any incorrect attributions (i.e. beliefs about the cause of a sensation) that the patient may be making to interpret their symptoms (e.g. that there must be something sinister to cause the pain, possibly cancer). A further example is the increased likelihood of an HIV-positive patient disclosing that they have sero-converted to a dentist who demonstrates sophisticated communication skills. Such skills include responding to the patient in a non-judgemental manner (Robinson et al. 1994).

BOX 6.2   ADVANTAGES OF GOOD
COMMUNICATION SKILLS

- Better diagnosis of your patients' problems
- Increased adherence of patients to your recommendations and advice
- Greater patient satisfaction with the care received
- Reduced patient complaints and litigation towards your treatment interventions.

The patient is more likely to accept the dentist's clinical decision concerning treatment if the dentist can match his or her own opinion with the patient's view. Such a matching procedure may be very straightforward as there is often very little discrepancy between the patient and dentist in explaining a particular symptom. It can be seen that in the majority of cases this procedure can be smoothly encountered and managed. However dissatisfaction and complaint are likely if the dentist does not discuss the patient's own view when it is quite different from the dentist. If the patient is satisfied with the explanation offered by the dentist – especially when it has been compared with the patient's own understanding of the problem – then fewer complaints will be made, the patient is likely to remain in treatment and adhere to recommendations to assist in the treatment regimen or self-care preventive approaches.

Components of communication skills

Two major aspects of communication skills are especially relevant to dental staff. They are information giving and the management of patient beliefs and associated emotions.

INFORMATION GIVING

An example illustrates the need to understand the importance of providing information. A dentist in general practice related his frustration with encouraging patients to improve their oral hygiene.

> I have a fair number of my patients whom I see every six months for a checkup examination and refer on to my hygienist for a prophylaxis. The levels of plaque appear not to change. I try to support my hygienist by explaining to the patient the need to maintain good oral hygiene. I think they simply forget what we say in the practice.

Although other factors are likely to be important (see Chapter 10) there has been considerable work specifically to understand how patients memorise (or not) health information given to them in the surgery or clinic (Ley 1988). The results of these studies may be summarised as follows:

- Patient educational level is not strongly related to the degree of recall. Other factors appear to be much more important, as listed below.
- There is a clear relationship between the number of statements presented to the amount recalled by the patient.
- Patients often forget what they are told. Some estimates put this figure as high as 60%.
- The level of the patient's medical knowledge is related to recall. This may be independent of educational experience or attainment.
- Very low or high levels of anxiety at the time of providing the information are predictive of poor recall.

- Those statements which are stressed as being important, and given to the individual first (primacy effect) in the patient–clinician encounter are more likely to be remembered. Statements at the end of the appointment are also likely to be remembered (recency effect).
- Statements that are 'chunked' together (i.e. explicit categorisation) aid recall. For example the dentist may say to a patient who has children when encouraging the patient to embark on a dental health promotion programme at home:

> I would like you to introduce three changes into your household, ...
> The *first* is to do with oral hygiene. I would like you to ensure that your children are in fact brushing their teeth as long as they say they are. In other words, can you be with them while they are brushing to supervise the time that they brush...
> *Second*, I would like you to try and manage their sweet eating so that they eat any sweets directly after their evening meal with you. This is better than having them spread out at various stages in the day...
> and *finally*, you'll remember what I said earlier about not being afraid to come and see me even if you think there is nothing wrong with your child's teeth. I am keen to see you and your children so that I can have a look at how your children are progressing and give you any advice I can to help.

Although verbal provision of information is the most common form of imparting dental and medical details of preventive procedures, description of illnesses, and treatment options there is a widespread adoption of other methods. These include giving written information in the form of leaflets or booklets. Although the design and production of a leaflet would appear to be a relatively straightforward endeavour, the experience of those who have made serious attempts to inform the public will say otherwise. From a patient's perspective the clinic staff member that thrusts a poorly prepared piece of photocopied text

to them presents a very mixed message. Careful attention must be paid to the design of such leaflets and realistic resources spent on producing a message that is likely to be read. To assist in preparing the content of the message a readability assessment is available known as the Flesch Formula. The formula computes a measure of reading ease and may be calculated by subtracting two quantities from an initial score of 207. The two quantities include firstly the average number of syllables per hundred words (W) multiplied by 0.85, and secondly the average number of words in a sentence (S) multiplied by 1.02. The full formula is:

$$\text{Reading ease} = 206.8 - 0.85W - 1.02S$$

Scores of greater than 80 denote a fairly easy script that should be read by over 90% of the adult population.

An example of this systematic approach has shown measurable benefits in a clinical setting. A leaflet was produced in Liverpool's regional dental teaching hospital to explain the third molar extraction procedure, the techniques employed and what the patient will experience together with possible complications (O'Neill, Humphris & Field 1996). Two experimental groups were included in the design of the study. The first group of patients was prompted to read the leaflet, whereas the second group was simply handed the leaflet at the initial examination procedure. Comparisons between knowledge change (as assessed from a multiple choice questionnaire given before and after treatment) were studied across the two groups and against two control groups (an 'attention' control group where patients were given a health education leaflet, and a standard care group with no written form of information provided). Results presented in Table 6.1 show that the prompted group made significant improvements in knowledge. The provision of a relevant leaflet alone gave measurable but smaller benefits. Further investigation of these patients' views determined that the relevant leaflet group were the most satisfied with their care. It would appear that for this operation the passive presentation of written information may be preferred rather than placing a demand on the patient to read supplied leaflets. Generalising from the results of this study

Table 6.1

Change in patient knowledge scores of third molar extraction (as assessed by MCQ)

Group[a]	n	Increase in knowledge
Third molar leaflet + prompt	16	2.19**
Third molar leaflet	18	1.78*
Control 1 (Dental health education leaflet)	16	0.13
Control 2 (standard care)	16	0.25

Notes:
** p < 001, * p < 06,
a All patients received verbal explanation of treatment procedure and possible complications. From O'Neill, Humphris & Field (1996)

to other conditions, such as surgical treatment for periodontal disease, would be risky. Using leaflets to prepare patients for satisfactory treatment of their periodontal disease may not be justified without a special study with this type of patient. Patients may prefer a more direct approach and receive all of their information from the dentist who is going to treat them. However it does illustrate the ability of the clinical researcher to investigate the benefits of a communicative intervention.

Other methods of providing information are being explored and systematically evaluated. Such work is evident particularly in the US, where practitioners are concerned to ensure that potential patients are fully aware of the risks associated with surgery (Ader et al. 1992). An example of this type of study has been reported by Ader who has developed a video approach to presenting patients with detailed information about the third molar extraction procedure, with special emphasis on the possible associated risks such as swelling, inflammation, infection and numbness. Patients are asked to view the programme and then complete a questionnaire to convey to the clinical team that they have understood the messages provided. With the advent of improved and 'easier-to-use' software there is likely to be an explosion of this type of preparatory material becoming available. Careful evaluation will be required to assess the benefits for patients; the potential is however encouraging as patients are more likely to

understand the health problems they encounter, and the treatment options available. It is nevertheless important to point out that the advent of new technologies that assist in the provision of information should be developed with clinicians and volunteer patients to produce packages which support the verbal exchanges between clinician and patient.

MANAGEMENT OF PATIENT BELIEFS ABOUT ILLNESS AND EMOTIONAL FACTORS

Apart from providing information, the other major aspect of communication skills is learning from patients whether they have any dental problems. The role is therefore reversed in that the dentist will be encouraging patients to provide information, not only of the facts related to any condition or problem they may wish to raise but also what they consider may have caused the problem (i.e. patient beliefs). Further information to be elicited from patients would be their feelings associated with the problem (e.g. anxiety about the invasiveness, or the cost, of any treatment required).

The setting or place in which the clinician meets the patient is very important. In ideal circumstances the dentist should be able to meet with a patient in a quiet, private room which is unlikely to be disturbed. These circumstances will give much greater opportunity for patients to broach difficult subject areas. Although there are excellent examples of a few practices where accommodation is sufficient to have a 'quiet' room for private discussions there is often insufficient space to introduce this facility. Even in cramped settings, however, such as in the surgery itself, there may be space for a conventional chair (rather than the dental chair) for the patient to be seated for an introductory discussion before any examination or treatment procedure takes place.

NON-VERBAL BEHAVIOUR

To encourage good communication between patient and dentist the use of non-verbal behaviour is essential – in fact it is impossible *not* to convey certain messages to patients. Difficulties can arise with patients when the dentist says one thing but then behaves in a totally contradictory manner which undermines what he or she has previously said. For example, the dentist may have asked the patient to relate what problems he has experienced since last seen. The question may well have been asked when the dentist was facing the patient, but after the question the dentist then turns to look on the shelf top behind the patient for his notes. The patient is unsure what to do, whether to say that he has been experiencing some minor pain in the lower arch, but then decides not to bother as the dentist seems not to be interested. This matching of non-verbal and verbal communication skills will ensure a consistent and unambiguous communication process.

Other non-verbal behaviours are listed in Box 6.3 and a description of a number of these is presented below.

BOX 6.3   COMPONENTS OF NON-VERBAL
COMMUNICATION

- Touch
- Proximity
- Posture and orientation
- Body movements and gestures
- Facial expression
- Gaze and eye contact
- Paralanguage
- General appearance.

Touch

Dentists are unique in many respects as they have to touch a sensitive part of the patient's body, the mouth. Touching behaviour is functional and has the purpose of completing various tasks associated with examination and treatment. Touch can be used as a means of comforting the patient, and also as a means of controlling, for example the dentist may gently place his hand to one side of the patient's face and gently press against the cheek of the patient to encourage him to turn his head. The manner in which this is done is critical so that the patient feels that he is not being coerced to embark on a procedure that he would

otherwise not sanction. The preferred method would be to assist the patient's head to move so that he is hardly aware of the influence as the movement of the hand coincides with the dentist's verbal request to move his head in the direction required. The consistency of verbal invitation and gentle direction should present a clear message to the patient.

Proximity

The dentist similarly has tacit permission to sit at close proximity to the patient – perhaps for some time – during a complex dental procedure. Social psychologists have observed that there appear to be three zones of proximity: intimate, personal and social consultative (Argyle, 1988). The intimate zone that includes actual body contact occupies a spot up to 18 inches from the body. This is the zone that dentists will operate in during examination and other clinical procedures. The majority of patients will accept that this very close proximity is essential for the dentist to do his job. The 'personal' zone for communicating with friends extends from 1–4 feet, whereas the 'social consultative' zone frequented by business acquaintances ranges from 4–12 feet. Strong evidence exists that we get closer to the people we like. Some patients may feel very uncomfortable and unable to inhibit the aversion that such close contact produces.

Posture and orientation

Orientation to the patient should be considered by the dentist especially when conversing about matters such as prevention of disease, maintenance of dental health and history taking. It is important for dentists to face their patients and observe the effects that their questions or advice may have. Important clues can be picked up by carefully observing the patient during this phase of the appointment. In addition it enables the patient to assess the dentist on a number of key qualities, such as warmth, genuineness and positive regard. Similar statements could also refer to the posture that the dentist adopts with the patient. Dentists who introduce themselves with their arms folded and the head tilted back will give an aloof impression.

Body movement

Hurried body movements should be avoided in close proximity to patients. Rapid movements increase uncertainty in the patient: a major component in the development and maintenance of dental anxiety (Lindsay & Jackson 1993).

Facial expression

Facial expression provides excellent confirmation of the meaning of information acquired verbally from the patient by the clinician and vice versa. In the dental situation however the patient's facial expressions are hampered by the fact that his mouth is often open for examination or treatment. With child patients, useful information can be drawn from the patient's eyes as an indicator of pain during a dental procedure (Rowland et al. 1989). Equally, the patient may not be able to determine from the dentist's face confirmatory details that support statements made verbally. This effect may not be great as the patient may still be able to assess whether the dentist is positively reinforcing them by the dentist's eyes – even if shielded by glasses, the patient can still observe them.

Gaze and eye contact

Duration of gaze and eye contact are powerful indicators of arousal. We tend to look more at the people we like. The converse is also true – that if we are aware that we are not being looked at then there is a covert message that individuals who avert their gaze are not interested in us.

Paralanguage

This component includes all those qualities of speech which do not involve the actual verbal content of the message, but which provide speech with an important extra dimension to the meaning of what a person is saying. Paralanguage includes the following elements: speed, inflexion, intonation, accent and volume.

Appearance

The clinician's appearance has traditionally been regarded as important in communicating a form of respect to the patient (Dickson, Hargie & Morrow 1989). The effect that the wearing of jewellery, flamboyant clothing, or unusual hair styles has on patient reactions is unresearched. A preliminary report that encouraged dentists to embark on more research on the type of clothing to be recommended to dental staff indicated, somewhat surprisingly, that the wearing of gloves was considered a mark of professionalism by respondents over the age of 40 years (Waddington 1996). Much of the above is knowledge that will have been acquired from magazines or television documentaries by students and clinicians independently of any formal teaching or training in research – however the strength of these effects is often underestimated.

Non-verbal behaviour (NVB) can in some circumstances replace the use of a verbal message, for example, a caring touch. As already mentioned the main function of NVB is to assist a verbal message and provide it with greater clarity or strength. The control of a communication process may be enhanced by the use of NVB. A great deal of NVB is expressed purely to ensure a smooth flow of utterances between the participants, e.g. to encourage each individual to take a turn. Patients can pick up messages from clinicians – such as the importance of the information being conveyed by the slow, deliberate delivery of a message – even if the patient does not understand the content of the message clearly. This is an example of a neglected area in non-verbal communication skills training: the use of 'paralanguage', which is defined as 'how something is said as opposed to what is said' (Dickson, Hargie & Morrow 1989). This means that vocalisations are studied in terms of their tone, pitch, volume, speed and accent. A low volume of voice in talking to children can be reinforcing and encourage attention to the message the dentist wishes to convey.

Case 6b   The importance of words in the clinical situation

Gender: Female   Age: 50   Occupation: Housewife

Referral: Secondary referral from one hospital unit to another

Problem: Edentulous following surgery to remove squamous cell carcinoma
Features: Distress at prospect of having to revisit dental hospital

A 50-year-old woman had been treated for a substantial oral facial tumour by extensive surgery and reconstruction, including bone grafts to the mandible to enable implants to be fitted once the tumour site had healed and settled down. She attended a specialist at a surgical unit and described her contact with the clinician as a very difficult experience. She vividly remembers the clinician at the outpatient clinic saying that the patient's mouth had been cleaned up as the 'dirt' had been removed in the initial surgery. The patient had been offended by the word 'dirt' and stated that this experience had been worse than the initial major surgery itself to remove the tumour and perform reconstruction.

VERBAL BEHAVIOUR

The importance of the appropriate selection of words is illustrated in the case above. That such a negative reaction was experienced by the patient should alert clinicians to the careful choice of words when describing an aspect of the patient's condition. This is vital when raising the issue of malignancy, so that any euphemisms, if they must be used, should be chosen carefully. When in doubt a helpful rule of thumb, supported by the literature, is to ask the patient. For example, if you feel cautious about mentioning a condition which you believe may have important repercussions, then it would be good practice to ask the patient how much he would prefer to learn from you about his condition. The large majority will opt for more extensive information, however there is a small but important minority who state a preference for not knowing about a serious or chronic disease.

The dental situation is somewhat unique in patient–clinician relationships. This uniqueness has often been picked up by comics and cartoonists who illustrate that the dentist may ask the patient an important question while the patient has his mouth open and filled with instruments, and is

therefore unable to make himself understood when attempting to speak. It is not unknown for some clinicians to use a rubber dam to prevent patients from speaking. Physical barriers to verbal communication may not work to the dentist's desired effect. The patient may feel frustrated, save questions to the end of the consultation, and so prolong the session. Modern dentistry, however, requires the dentist to embark on procedures in which the patient will be unable to talk. The noise of the high and low speed drill and the aspirator as well as the physical presence of these and other dental instruments will make speaking very difficult. Devising methods for patients to indicate discomfort or their wish to take a 'breather' will be discussed in the next chapter. Clinicians should therefore adapt their communication skills to various phases of the appointment in order to compensate for those occasions when exchange of two-way communication is difficult. It could be argued that the dentist has more responsibility to pace the communication process than his colleagues in general medical practice.

Audio recording of clinical sessions in dental practice has revealed a relatively clear structure and has been referred to as the 'dental consultation' (Wanless & Hollaway 1994). Thirty general dental practitioners were audiotaped with 132 adolescent patients aged 10–17 years. The elements of the consultation are listed in Table 6.2. Not all the stages were apparent in every meeting with a patient. For instance, only 56% of consultations included a verbal greeting, although the dentists, may well have adopted a non-verbal method to introduce themselves. Explanations were often given (49% of consultations) but opportunity for patients to express their feelings (14%) or involving patients in decision making (12%) were less likely. An omission noted by the authors was the lack of quantifying non-verbal behaviour that could be collected through videotape. A broad three-stage consultation process has been identified in the dental interview comprising: Opening, Examination and Treatment, and Closing (Newton 1995). The term Closing is preferable to Dismissal. However more instructive is the term recently employed to describe the final stage of the consultation process, namely Sustaining. With the patient, the dentist reviews the maintenance of his dental

Table 6.2

Frequency of stages in 132 dental consultations by 30 dentists (presented as percentages)

Stage	Consultations
Greeting	56
Preliminary chat	48
Preliminary explanation	19
Business	100
Summary	4
Health education	34
Dismissal	30

From Wanless & Hollaway (1994)

health by negotiating a further visit or recommendation for improved oral hygiene practices (Gibson et al. 1997). Further studies are required within the dental context. We need to know in more detail what communication procedures are being used in other age groups and with particular types of patient and dentist.

It is important that the dentist is aware of the various stages in an interaction between patient and dentist during an appointment. Even when an appointment may last only a few minutes, as in an examination, the processes that occur are likely to be recognisable within this structure. Initiating and opening skills are important to start the communication process. Studies that have observed junior medical staff have noted that their introductions to patients are poor with many not even using their names (Maguire 1986) or indicating the purpose of the meeting. Results from other health professions are no better with patients finding it difficult to remember the name of the person they met. Effort expended by the dentist in the 'greeting, meeting and seating' of the patient is warranted and has been summarised by Hargie, Saunders & Dickson (1987).

1. Arrange the environment in a co-operative or 'user-friendly' fashion.
2. Appropriate greeting behaviour which may involve standing and meeting the patient at the door, smiling, engaging in eye contact, using 'non-task comments' (such as discussing the weather briefly or commenting on a holiday the patient may have had), and offering a seat.
3. Motivating the patient by indicating interest, giving full attention and showing concern.

4. Checking various details with the patient such as the name and address, introducing oneself and the dental surgery assistant, stating the purpose of the visit, obtaining the patient's expectations and then outlining what is going to happen.

A critical part of the verbal communication skills process is that the dentist must spend some time listening to the patient. Some authors stress that this skill is the most important of all. The term 'active listening' has been applied to illustrate that this means more than simply keeping quiet and letting the patient speak. However, some improvement in the communication skills of health professionals would be seen by purely practising the latter, that is, passive listening. Active listening involves taking notes and analysing what the patient is saying 'on the fly' by examining the content of what the patient is saying and seeing if this matches his non-verbal behaviour, plus interjecting occasionally to clarify a point (which improves the quality of the interaction in most cases, as the patient is made aware that the dentist is taking an interest) and reflecting.

REFLECTION

Use of reflection is helpful when a patient relates how he feels about an event, or symptom, and the dentist responds by repeating how the patient felt, for example:

Patient: This tooth at the front I chipped quite badly. I can't feel any difference except that it seems from when I touch the tooth with my tongue, it is as if a huge chunk has gone from it. I'm wondering if the nerve will die like it did with my friend. The tooth went all black. I thought she looked terrible. She had to have the tooth taken out. I don't want to end up like that.

Dentist: It sounds to me as if you are very worried about losing that tooth.

The use of reflection is a key skill that requires practice to perform well. It is rewarding for patients as they report that the clinician really understood what they were saying. Clinicians also find the employment of the skill a challenge as they have to listen to their patients closely to be able to summarise and reflect the details of what the patient has told them. It is important, however, not to attempt to interpret what a patient has said in terms of feelings or emotion unless the patient has explicitly made this clear in the verbal exchange. Reflection however is a good method of checking with the patient that you have understood them. It allows the patient to correct the clinician if the details have not been reflected correctly or the patient wishes to change his story. Sometimes the process of relating a symptom, an important event or sharing a problem can shed a new light for the patient who then has a second chance to express himself. The procedure for patients is intrinsically rewarding, and the dentist gains by obtaining a much clearer picture of the patient's concerns. The act of rehearsing the information that the patient has given them will improve recall of the patient in future meetings and encourage a stronger patient–dentist relationship.

ASSERTION

Other skills requiring care and careful training are the use of assertion, pacification and confrontation. Assertiveness is a skill that may occasionally be required if patients or other members of the healthcare team make undue demands which are beyond your responsibility to provide because of unrealistic time pressures, cost or inadequate training. One procedure that may be adopted (known as empathic assertion) is simple in theory but in practice is difficult to achieve without rehearsal and discussion with experienced trainers. The procedure is to reflect what the person has requested and acknowledge what they must be feeling in order to demonstrate that you are aware of their demand and what it means to them. However the next stage is to say a firm 'no' to the request, saying that it is not possible. If an excuse is given then this is repeated simply should the person making the unreasonable request attempt to refute the excuse (broken record technique). Assertiveness skills would rarely be used with patients – in fact it is much more likely that patients should be taught these skills. This does raise the issue of power (already discussed in Chapter 2) where clinicians must closely inspect their relationship with their patients in order that their

clinical decision making abilities do not introduce an abuse of power. Although it is regarded as important to provide patients with ways to influence decisions (sometimes termed empowerment – see Chapter 10) in some instances, albeit fairly rare, patients are able to encourage their clinician to embark on an unnecessary procedure, for example general anaesthesia for a routine examination.

HOSTILITY

The prevention of an aggressive outburst from a patient (or for that matter a colleague) requires a very different approach. Non-threatening behaviour in response to threat – becoming passive and extremely pleasant – is important to gain time to encourage the possible assailant to calm down and become aware of his anger and hostile feelings. In situations where patients become aggressive it is important to try and stay calm, maintaining a reasonable distance but not too far away, being honest, and helping the patient to feel he has a choice in the predicament in which he finds himself. Do not threaten or interrupt his speech (words are better than violent outburst), do not block his path should he wish to leave, do not take offence at his speech and do not touch him as this may be misconstrued as an offensive action. Negotiating and bargaining may be required in order to allow yourself to exit the situation and call for assistance.

CONFRONTATION

Occasionally the use of confrontation may be required when, for instance, a patient presents you with information which is clearly not verified by other information to which you have access. The term confrontation should be interpreted with care as it does not mean the use of an aggressive approach, but rather helping the patient recognise that you are aware of a discrepancy in the facts you have about him and you are confused about how to proceed. By appealing for his assistance there is a greater likelihood that he will supply you with a more coherent explanation. An example of this would be the emergency patient insisting that you remove a number of teeth at once because he is experiencing intense pain in a quadrant of the mouth. On inspection of the area you can find very little evidence of pathology. Your decision to intervene should be delayed until you are clearer about the nature of the symptoms experienced by the patient, duration, remedies previously tried, advice already received, and the patient's view of the cause of the pain: to say bluntly that you will not do anything is inappropriate. Discussion with the patient about the nature of pain, the irreversibility of extractions, the patient's fears about what the pain may indicate (e.g. a member of the patient's family may have suffered orofacial cancer and presented with similar symptoms) may help to resolve a confusing and demanding situation.

The use of communication skills when treatment complications arise

Reports put the number of official complaints made by patients in the form of a legal claim as less than 2%, however the cost to the clinician and the patient is high even with this low incidence rate. It is recognised that there are four factors which can help to avert complaints when things go wrong with treatment (the four Ss):

- Speed
- Sympathy
- Satisfaction
- 'Sorry'.

Each of these responses requires a substantial use of communication skills (Matthews, 1995).

Speed. If problems occur during the treatment procedure, such as a pulp becoming exposed during cavity preparation, the patient should be informed and options discussed. Information about various options should be given and checks made with the patient that the dentist's explanation has been understood. If the patient identifies that a problem has arisen and contacts the dental surgery, it is important that the dentist attempts to speak to the patient in person. The patient will feel that his grievance has been taken seriously. Other members of the dental team must be informed so as to be receptive when the patient next makes contact. When patients complain it is essential to allow

them time to explain what they understand the problem to be and how they feel about it. Only then should the member of staff attempt to assist explanation and discussion of how to proceed. Arguments or competitive viewpoints are, however, likely to inflame at this initial stage.

Sympathy: The use of reflection, for example

> *Dentist*:   This must be quite a shock for you, and I can understand that you are very upset by what has happened.
>
> *Patient*:   Well at least you recognise that I am very upset about what has happened.

This type of statement will help to convey to the patient that you have listened to his problem and are appreciative of how he feels. Simply being sympathetic in this manner can often achieve diffusion of a great deal of distress and anger that patients can sometimes feel.

Satisfaction. In order to make amends the surgery staff need to allow the patient to feel that his or her view has been listened to. Alternative treatment avenues need to be discussed and great care taken to ensure that any further appointments that are required are checked with staff. It must be ensured that punctuality and the necessary instruments and materials can be prepared in readiness. All of these areas will require a good communication system between members of staff in the clinic or practice.

'Sorry'. The person who is responsible for the clinical care of the patient should apologise in person. In the UK, an expression of regret would not be regarded as an admission of liability, although if you are in doubt you should check with your defence union. However, patients do expect to receive some apologetic explanation of the error that occurred.

In his book, Matthews presents a case where a dentist extracted a loose upper deciduous tooth from an 11-year-old girl using local anaesthesia (Matthews 1995 p 106). The extracted tooth slipped from the forceps and dropped into the pharynx. The dentist explained immediately to the parents what had happened, and then accompanied the patient to hospital following a call to A&E to warn of their arrival. The tooth was removed following bronchoscopy. The dentist stayed with the family throughout. According to Matthews, the dentist averted a claim because of his skill in communicating speedily, as well as the care and concern that he was able to express.

To protect patients from treatment they would prefer not to have and to prevent dentists from being accused of negligence or battery it is vital that informed consent is obtained (see Box 6.4). To obtain consent to conduct a procedure for a child requires substantial care and attention. In effect there are three parties involved in a complex relationship: the interests and responsibilities of the dentist, the rights and freedoms of the child and the responsibilities and autonomy of the parents all have to be safeguarded. The current emphasis of consent appears to be shifting from parent to child. Many children are entirely comfortable in deferring to their parent to make a decision about treatment. The majority of adolescents have however been shown able and willing to make decisions about their own health-care treatments, especially if there are possibly serious implications should complications arise (Scherer & Reppucci 1988). You are advised to ensure that adolescents are brought into discussions concerning their treatment. Young children who have deferred their decision to their parents should have the procedures explained to them. It is important that you are vigilant and study the professional press to keep abreast with new developments in this area.

BOX 6.4   FEATURES OF INFORMED CONSENT

Three features of consent in the dental context are listed. Consent should be obtained, preferably in writing, before a treatment procedure is started.

1. The patient needs to be told about the treatment procedure. The information should include details of both the benefits and the risks. Be prepared to discuss even very small risks. More recent evidence shows that a sizeable proportion of patients are keen to know about serious risks as low as one in a million. The patient should be able to understand the information you provide, therefore follow the guidelines of good information giving:
   - Use short words and sentences
   - Avoid jargon
   - Check that the patient understands your message (do this more than once during your explanation)
   - Ensure that you ask the patient for any questions they might have
   - Supplement your verbal information with written leaflets (see earlier in this chapter).
2. Patient consent must be given voluntarily. Do not exert subtle pressure on the patient. When patients consent to a procedure, ensure that it is their own decision.
3. The patient should be competent to make the decision. That is, the clinician has to make a judgement that the patient is capable of understanding the information given, that he or she is able to make a choice and can communicate this choice to you. (Scherer & Reppucci 1988)

Although consent typically refers to surgical treatment, the same rules apply when consenting patients enter a Randomised Clinical Trial to test a new procedure or drug. Advice should be sought from your local Research Ethical Committee as additional information would need to be supplied. For example, if patients decided not to enter the study, reassurance must be given that they would still receive the standard high quality care they can reasonably expect from a health service provider. (Scherer & Reppucci 1988)

Communication skills training

Many dental schools are now introducing communication skills training programmes to help students learn some of the building blocks in the communication process. There has been a rapid growth in this form of training in medicine and interest is growing in the dental field. Undoubtedly, there is overlap with the teaching received in clinical skills training. However, the development of clinical skills has often been so demanding that the emphasis on communication skills can be minimal. Hence the need for a special programme for dental students is commended, especially as the tasks required of the dentist, as has been argued earlier, is unique in that close physical contact is nearly always made with the patient. The transfer of newly practised skills from the group room to the clinic and eventually to the surgery is not a smooth process. Students require a clear rationale for the behaviour being advocated, and support from supervisors and senior staff to help maintain these skills. An approach that includes skills practice (that is, actions that are referred to as behavioural approaches) and, for instance, assessment of the advantages and disadvantages of various alternative skills available (i.e. assessment that requires thinking processes and is often referred to as cognitive approaches) is being developed to assist in the generalisation of this teaching beyond the class-room. The use of 'cognitive scripts' becomes more sophisticated as training continues. Cognitive scripts refer not only to the words that might be used in a certain situation, but also how they would be said and what posture, timing, tone of voice should be adopted. These 'scripts' help the acquired skills from being dismissed as not integral to the behavioural repertoire of the developing clinician (Kinderman & Humphris 1995).

Use of communication skills with other members of the health team

Some of the skills employed with patients described above are appropriate for use with colleagues in the dental healthcare team. However, additional skills of team working are essential for modern dentists to acquire in order to assist the practice or clinic within which they are working and to provide the highest quality care available. The skills required by team members centre around issues of clinical practice, continuing education and administration. Barriers to multiprofessional communication in teams can arise through:

- Lack of availability of members of the team
- Evaluation (usually negative) instead of specific two-way feedback made regularly
- Poor consultation throughout the team
- Competition and rivalry between professions
- Inadequate record-keeping
- Lack of guidelines, policies and protocols
- Exclusion of team members in decision making.

Many of the barriers listed above are obvious. However, the use of evaluation – which is so important in assessing the effectiveness of new treatments or health education interventions (see Chapter 10) – must be introduced very carefully for a team to work well with each other and prevent splits occurring. Feedback which affirms the work produced by team members that is specific to tasks completed can cement the team together. Occasions when a task has gone awry are easier to raise with the team member concerned if regular factual feedback is maintained. In addition the issue of competition between disciplines, professions and individuals within teams is common and potentially very damaging for patient care, especially in senior staff. Rivalries can persist for years and efforts to defuse these at an early stage are a formidable challenge to the team management.

To improve your communications with your colleagues in the team who are from the same profession, the following suggestions are made:

- Prepare a policy statement (also known as a mission statement) for the team
- Have regular meetings and consult staff
- Ensure senior staff are available for consultation
- Provide support and advice to staff
- Give orientation to new staff
- Delegate tasks to all members of the team.

To encourage team members from different professions to work well together in promoting health and healthcare, certain communication strategies may be required (Fielding 1995). In order to share clinical work for instance, development programmes in collaborative practice are to be encouraged. These may for instance include expanded roles for certain staff categories (such as dental therapists) where legal responsibilities for patients allow. Shared care plans with joint review procedures can be instituted after consultation and joint decisions to embark on change have been achieved. Integrated record-keeping across team members would improve communication among the disciplines and assist directly in the care of patients. For dentists, a period of training may be required to develop a maturity that can accept a more collaborative approach as opposed to dominance of other staff.

Other face-to-face communication issues that are beyond the scope of this introductory text to explore in depth are listed in summary form in Box 6.5. These have been drawn together from general dental practitioners.

BOX 6.5 FURTHER COMMUNICATION CHALLENGES FOR THE CLINICIAN

- **The uncommunicative or secretive patient**
  The patient may be withdrawn (due to depression), naturally shy or very anxious. Some patients attending their dentist may be involved in behaviour or have conditions they feel guilty or embarrassed about, e.g. drug taking, incontinence, disabilities. An understanding and non-judgemental presentation by the clinician is an important prerequisite in assisting these patients through their dental treatment.
- **The 'enmeshed' family**
  Occasionally parents (or step-parents) become very protective of the children they regard as their prime responsibility. Children may respond with uncertainty in how to accept dental procedures that they believe may be uncomfortable. Parents who are very close to their children become concerned when they sense their child's uncertainty. This pattern may develop and be maintained making it very difficult for the dentist to proceed adopting a standard approach. Good listening skills are important in allowing the participants (child and family) to express concerns. The likely result in due course is a greater acceptability of treatment procedures.

- **The overfamiliar patient**
  Dental staff are advised to present as 'warm and friendly' and engage in non-dental topics of discussion. Clear boundaries are required therefore so that dental staff may maintain appropriate relationships with patients and their relatives. Difficulties can arise when incremental liberties may be taken by a patient over a series of visits when the dental member of staff finds it difficult to assert that the patient behaviour in question (for example, inappropriate touching such as deliberately brushing against a member of staff) is not acceptable.
- **The patient with communication difficulties**
  Patients who have problems in making themselves understood include those from other cultures and those with disabilities. Problems of hearing or speech can interfere greatly and the clinician must attempt to try and understand the patient. This will be assisted by staying with the patient and trying various approaches. Just speaking with raised volume does not help and can embarrass. Try using other methods, modes of speech, writing, other people (an interpreter). Once some contact has been successfully made try not to assume you have got the point of the patient's communication without checking first. Ingenuity is often required with the assistance of relatives or friends. Be careful not to ignore the patient when asking for help from a relative.

References

Ader D, Seibring A, Bhaskar P, Melamed B 1992 Information seeking and interactive videodisc preparation for third molar extraction. Journal of Oral Maxillofacial Surgery 50:27–31

Argyle M 1988 Bodily communication (2nd edn.) London: Routledge

Audit Commission 1993 What's the matter? London: HMSO

Boyle C M 1970 Differences between patients' and doctors' interpretations of some common medical terms. British Medical Journal 2:286–289

Corah N L, O'Shea R M, Bissell G D et al. 1988 The dentist–patient relationship: perceived dentist behaviours that reduce patient anxiety and increase satisfaction. Journal of the American Dental Association *116*:73–76

Dickson D A, Hargie O, Morrow N C 1989 Communication skills training for health professionals. London: Chapman & Hall

Fielding R 1995 Clinical communication skills. Hong Kong: Hong Kong University Press

Gibson B, Drennan J, Hanna S, Freeman R 1997 Routine dentalling and the six monthly check-up. British Society of Dental Research, Brighton

Hargie O, Saunders C, Dickson D 1987 Social skills in inter-personal communication (2nd edn.) London: Croom Helm

Kinderman P, Humphris G M 1995 The role of cognitive schemata in clinical communication skills teaching. Medical Education *29*:436–442

Ley P 1988 Communicating with patients. London: Chapman & Hall

Lindsay S J E, Jackson C 1993 Fear of routine dental treatment in adults: its nature and management. Psychology and Health *8*(2,3):165–174

Maguire P 1986 Social skills training for health professionals. In: Holin C, Trower P (eds.) Handbook of social skills training. London: Croom Helm

Matthews J B R 1995 Risk management in dentistry. Oxford: Wright

Newton T 1995 Dentist/patient communication: a review. Dental Update *22*:118–122

O'Neill P, Humphris G M, Field E A 1996 The use of an information leaflet for patients undergoing wisdom tooth removal. British Journal of Oral & Maxillofacial Surgery *34*:331–334

Robinson P, Zakrzewska J, Maini M, Williamson D, Croucher R 1994 Dental visiting behaviour and experiences of men with HIV. British Dental Journal *176*:175–179

Rowland A, Lindsay S J E, Winchester L, Zarkowska E 1989 A study of facial expressions of pain and fear during dental treatment and their relationship to disruptive behaviour and reports of pain and fear. Journal of Paediatric Dentistry *5*:115–120

Scherer D, Reppucci N 1988 Adolescents' capacities to provide voluntary informed consent. Law and Human Behaviour *12*(2):123–141

Waddington T 1996 MRI Update: The effect of dentist attire on patient perceptions of skill, caring and professionalism. British Dental Journal *180*:86–87

Wanless M B, Hollaway P J 1994 An analysis of audio-recordings of general dental practitioners' consultations with adolescent patients. British Dental Journal *177*:94–98

7

Managing patient anxiety

Dental anxiety is probably the major management difficulty for dentists and has therefore attracted considerable interest. Moderate dental anxiety is very common. Sixty-eight per cent of respondents in the UK 1988 Adult Dental Health Survey moderately or strongly agreed with the statement 'I'm nervous with some kinds of dental treatment'. At higher levels of dental anxiety patients miss appointments and delay checkups. Fear of the dentist was rated by 45% of the dentate adults in the survey as the most important barrier to dental care (Todd & Lader 1991). Other factors considered in the survey, namely image of the dentist and cost of treatment were rated as considerably less important, i.e. 22% for both factors. The purpose of this chapter therefore is to provide an overview of some of the major themes and translate them into a practical guide of assessment and possible therapeutic approaches. Although the emphasis will tend to be on practice the principal findings that are prominently discussed among researchers will be highlighted. It is hoped therefore that you will be introduced to current issues in what is a complex and fascinating field.

The terms dental anxiety and fear require some explanation as they are in effect used interchangeably by many who discuss or write about dental anxiety. Dental phobia is a specific condition that prevents individuals from visiting the dentist but also affects their view of themselves and how they socialise. Descriptions of these terms are presented in Boxes 7.1 to 7.3.

For the purposes of this chapter the term anxiety will be principally used as this is the most common experience. However when dealing with strong, though transitory reactions the term fear will be applied.

BOX 7.1   ANXIETY

Anxiety refers to a hypothetical psychological construct which is:
- Anticipatory
- Associated to a specific event (but not always)
- Aversive
- Unpleasant to experience; and
- Takes time to dissipate.

Three components are helpful in explaining anxiety.
1. Physiological and somatic sensations, for example:
   - Breathlessness
   - Perspiration
   - Palpitations
   - Feelings of unease.

2. Cognitive features (that is, how changes occur in thinking processes), for example:
   - Interference of concentration
   - A focusing of attention sometimes known as hypervigilance
   - Inability to remember certain events while anxious
   - Imagining the worst that could happen.

3. Behavioural reactions, for example:
   - Avoidance, i.e. the postponing of a dental appointment, or requesting to have all dental treatment conducted in a single session.
   - Escape from the situation which precipitates the anxiety.

BOX 7.2   FEAR

Fear overlaps with the anxiety construct but emphasises a more biological response. Someone who experiences fear will not necessarily be anticipating a negative event, – their response will occur at the moment the unpleasant event (e.g. pain) occurs. In a sense the fear response is a valuable one, in that it produces a protective 'fight or flight' response. That is, the individual who experiences fear (and the physiological reactions can be magnified relative to anxiety), usually in response to a clear unpleasant stimulus, selects whether to engage in defence ('fight') or makes a hasty retreat ('flight'). Either way the fear response can be quickly resolved and dissipated. In this sense fear may be seen more positively as the individual is very often clear what precipitated the fear reaction.

A panic reaction is a special type of fear, sometimes regarded as a 'fear of fear itself'. The individual who suffers a panic reaction is acutely aware of the physiological sensations within his body and certain symptoms he experiences act to trigger a full-blown fear reaction. This experience may well be more common in dental patients than has hitherto been realised and will be discussed later in the chapter.

BOX 7.3   DENTAL PHOBIA

Dental phobia shares features of anxiety and fear. It is an unfortunate term as the person who is considered to be dentally phobic can become labelled, although dental phobia may be regarded as an extreme reaction to dental stimuli. It shares features that are apparent with other well known phobias such as spider and rat phobias. These include:

- A highly developed avoidance response
- Sufferers are unable to explain their reactions
- Embarrassment and shame.

The social consequences of dental phobia have been neglected. Sufferers are not able to talk about their difficulties easily because they feel their problem is ridiculous. The clinician who attempts to inform a phobic patient of the reasons for the phobia, and says that it could be controlled if the patient only tried hard enough is likely to frustrate the patient. Of course this assumes the dentist comes into contact with individuals with dental phobia – the majority of sufferers will not be able to enter the surgery door.

Causes of dental anxiety

There is a great deal of interest in the development of dental anxiety. The principal factor currently employed to help explain the cause of dental anxiety is a traumatic experience while at the dentist. A substantial amount of research – although nearly all retrospective – has shown the high incidence of unpleasant events during a dental appointment and a causal link with dental anxiety. Other factors have been implicated and these principal explanations are listed in Box 7.4.

BOX 7.4   CAUSES OF DENTAL ANXIETY

- Traumatic experiences
  Single event (Flashbulb memories)
  Repetitive events
- Vicarious learning
  Friends
  Parents
  Media (e.g. TV, radio, film, magazines and newspapers)
- Preparedness
- Personality.

The most obvious traumatic experience at the dentist is sudden unexpected pain during a dental procedure. In a large study with adults from Norway ($n = 3670$) about 60% reported having had at least one very painful experience, and of these just over 5% rated dental treatment to be generally very painful (Vassend 1993). Unfortunately dentists cannot always control sudden pain. The most anxiety-provoking procedure at the dentist has been reported to be the local anaesthetic (Humphris, Morrison & Lindsay 1995). Studies examining the effectiveness of local anaesthetics (LA) show that at least 10% of locals fail, and these estimates rely on the dentists themselves assessing patients' experience – the failure rate could therefore well be higher. Among a US sample of university employees 49% could remember one or more LA failures while having dental treatment. More recently, when seven dental practitioners from the UK rated LA administrations for pain and related their scores to their patients it was found that there was good correspondence between professional and patient ratings. In addition it was found that 93% of LAs were rated as comfortable by both patient and dentist together. However, this favourable result may have been expected. The dentists were a self-selected group who were likely to spend considerable effort in providing pain-free injections.

Pain from other procedures such as scaling, which traditionally does not merit local anaesthesia, may feature as unpleasant enough to encourage a fear reaction. It can be argued then that the likelihood of patients experiencing completely pain-free dentistry is very low: a difficulty is understanding, however, whether pain experience can be responsible for all dental fears and anxiety. Fig. 7.1 shows how a painful stimulus at the dentist which produces a fearful reaction becomes paired with a hitherto neutral stimulus such as the dentist holding a syringe. The next occasion the patient sees the dentist with a syringe the patient experiences a strong fear reaction even though the dentist has not given an injection. This process is known as classical conditioning after the original work of Pavlov, the Russian physiologist. This suggested explanation for anxiety development does not, however, explain why people who experience an event of considerable pain at the dentist do not always develop dental anxiety.

A possible answer to this question has been proposed by Davey as an adjunct to the classical conditioning explanation. He found that students reported less anxiety if they had received a number

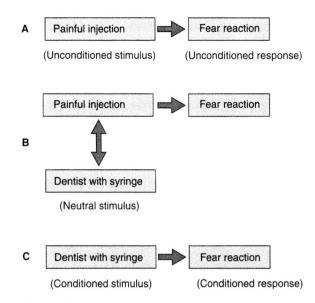

Fig.7.1 Example of classical conditioning. A: before conditioning a painful injection would elicit a fearful patient reaction. B: during conditioning the neutral stimulus of the dentist with the syringe is linked together with the painful injection. C: after conditioning the dentist with a syringe will encourage a fear reaction.

of painless treatments before a painful dental experience when compared to those without the positive visits before the traumatic episode (Davey 1989). This result supports what is known as the *latent inhibition hypothesis*. That is, if an unpleasant event is preceded by a number of positive experiences in the same setting then anxiety does not occur. An important study that asked children about their dental anxiety at nine years of age and then three years later when they were twelve, gives some additional and surprising findings (Murray, Liddell & Donohue 1989). Children who had not received invasive treatment during the three-year period were significantly more anxious than those who had. Regular attenders who had received invasive treatment had no change in their dental anxiety. What may have happened with these children is that regular experience of dental treatment (which was non-traumatic) prevented dental anxiety increasing. Clinicians have to appreciate that dental anxiety, treatment experience and regularity of attendance are associated in ways that need careful study. Personal assessment of patients is crucial for the clinician to understand how they feel when they attend the dental surgery.

Patients report other adverse experiences apart from pain. Dentists who continue a treatment procedure when the patient is attempting to stop the dentist (by raising an arm or attempting to say something) can generate great distress. This is more likely if the dentist has explained that the patient may stop them at any time during the procedure. Other patients report being humiliated by a dentist who berates them (maybe unwittingly) for not attending sooner. Dentists often feel that earlier treatment would have saved the patient's teeth from extraction or extensive restoration. Unfortunately these statements are often interpreted as criticism and therefore punishing for the patient. These often vivid experiences can hold a special place in the memories of individuals as already mentioned in Chapter 2. Recent work by psychologists with people who have experienced trauma in other settings apart from dentistry (for example, scenes of violent crime, or tragedy) have put forward interesting explanations as to why certain vivid events tend to exercise an enormous hold on the individual. Such people have the capacity to relive the original traumatic experience with extraordinary clarity. One such patient was noted as saying:

> I can remember the sound of the drill and wishing him to stop the drilling. The pain was unbearable as the local didn't work properly as it should have done. What gets me even now was how the second hand moving around the clock on the far wall of the surgery shook every second it moved around the dial. The wallpaper was clean around one side of the clock where someone must have moved the clock slightly when cleaning or something.

Such memories are known as *Flashbulb Memories* (FM) and are held in store ready for easy retrieval owing to the special way that these memories are 'encoded' in the brain (Conway 1995). The formation of an FM is reliant on a number of factors which may all be satisfied in the dental situation. That is, the traumatic event must have been a surprise, have consequences for the patient, produce a strong emotional reaction and rate as important to the individual.

The *vicarious experience* (that is, where the individual hears from another about their traumatic experience) has been put forward as another way in which dental anxiety may develop.

Although this route appears very plausible it is difficult to demonstrate. It does have obvious application in understanding the development of dental anxiety in some children who are relatively naïve about dentistry and pick up 'gory details' from playground stories. Some children may develop dental anxiety from parents or grandparents. Once again it is difficult to pin down how strong the influence of parents may be, particularly when many parents are aware that anxiety can be 'transferred' to their child, and as a consequence some parents are very careful not to discuss their fears in front of their child. There is some evidence that in young children with little prior experience of their own of dentistry that the parent's dental anxiety may be implicated in their child's view of dentistry.

Mixed approaches to developing anxiety are of course possible. People who have experienced a dentally traumatic experience and become dentally anxious may selectively attend to others in conversations and the media about dental misfortunes: this reinforces their negative experience and hence makes trying to cope with their anxiety more difficult. The evidence for selective attention, such as a bias towards gazing, for instance, at pictures of situations in a dental practice was not related to the degree of dental anxiety rated by potential patients (de Jongh et al. 1995b).

Personality has been a serious contender over the years in helping to explain why some individuals develop dental anxiety. Those who favour this view regard persons who develop anxiety to be prone to reacting more strongly to novel environments and procedures, or be more sensitive. This 'negative reactivity' may be due to specific underlying aspects of the individual's psychological makeup. The evidence of personality acting in this way is far from strong (Horst & Wit 1993). The link with general anxiety (sometimes referred to as 'free-floating anxiety') appears to be fairly weak (Moore, Brodsgard & Birn 1991), although there will always be cases where individuals present with high levels of dental anxiety who are also anxious to a range of other environments such as hospitals and, public spaces. What may be fruitful is to examine whether some people are vulnerable to unpleasant experiences. For instance psychology students who were afraid of the dentist were also afraid of pain, mutilation and showed some features of agoraphobia (Vignehsa et al. 1990).

A further possible explanation of why people develop dental anxiety is that they are in some way innately predisposed to be anxious about the dentist. As broached by Kent and Croucher (1998) this may appear far-fetched until it is recognised that some phobias are much more common than would be expected from the real threat that they pose – so that snake and spider phobias are common but a phobia to busy roads and motorways is not. There may therefore be some predisposition to being anxious about the dentist. This idea is described by psychologists as *preparedness*. We are predisposed to be sensitive towards certain stimuli. This susceptibility encourages learning to become afraid in the dental setting. This phenomenon may be a result of genetic inheritance or natural selection. It should not perhaps surprise us that some individuals develop insurmountable fears, when lying on their backs with sharp instruments in their mouths.

The significance of the mouth as a special area of concern has been highlighted for many years and may be termed a psychodynamic explanation for dental anxiety (Freeman 1998). There are many anecdotal reports from dream analyses and from clinical case histories of people who attach dramatic significance to the loss of their teeth or to the prospect of dentists treating their dentition. Verifying the concepts raised for empirical testing are far from straightforward and attempts to understand dental anxiety via this approach has therefore tended to diminish. A careful and assiduous use of audio and videotaped material should allow a closer examination of surface and deeper processes via discourse analysis (see Chapter 11) providing the ability to critically test psychodynamic approaches to understanding and treating the dentally anxious patient.

Assessment of dental anxiety

The assessment of dental anxiety may be split into three components (Table 7.1):

- Physiological
- Self-report
- Behavioural.

The physiological measures provide reassuring 'hard' data in the form of continuous monitoring of heart rate or some other indicator such as Galvanic Skin Response (GSR). These measures suffer, however, from the expense, complexity and recording capacity of the instrumentation. People may be influenced by the fact that they are being monitored, although this is usually discounted by taking resting levels of the parameters to be measured under relaxed conditions. This preparatory recording provides a baseline to interpret the data collected. In addition, the changes detected by these instruments may be due to other emotional effects such as hostility (towards having to wear electrodes) or embarrassment at being closely monitored when the individual feels that they cannot refuse.

Behavioural observation scales are a popular method of collecting data especially in very young children who may find questionnaires difficult to comprehend. A number of scales have been developed and include a simple four point scale for clinicians to score the overall disruptiveness of the session (Frankl, Shiere & Fogels 1962). The four

Table 7.1		
Advantages and disadvantages of various assessments of dental anxiety		
	Advantages	**Disadvantages**
Physiological (examples: Galvanic skin response; Palmar sweat index; Heart rate)	Standardised 'Hard' data	Questionable validity Instrumentation problems
Self-report (example: Corah's Dental Anxiety Scale)	Easily obtained data Flexible Ability to assess variety of aspects (e.g. trait and state)	Validity assumed rather than formally tested Difficult to measure during procedure itself
Behavioural (example: Frankl's Behaviour Rating Scale)	Objective	Difficult to define categories of behaviour Time consuming to score Technical problems with correct sampling of behaviour

---

BOX 7.5   GALVANIC SKIN RESPONSE

Electrodes placed on the patient's skin surface, especially where there are many skin pores such as the palm of the hand, will detect fluctuations in current between the two electrodes that coincides with significant events such as a loud noise or flash of light. The information supplied gives an accurate record of the sweat gland activity on the skin surface. Such changes in the recorded electrical potential give an indication of a person's emotional response to events such as sitting in the dental chair, preparing for an injection, having a filling. The electrical activity can be displayed on a screen (e.g. visual display unit) for viewing to act as biofeedback. Patients can use the information presented during dental procedures to attempt to reduce their GSR and consequently adopt a more relaxed approach.

---

points range from definitely negative (refusal of treatment) to definitely positive (good rapport and interested in procedures). The two middle points are named slightly negative and slightly positive, and are less easy to distinguish. Strictly speaking this may not be an anxiety scale as Lindsay has stated that children who develop unco-operative behaviour in the dental surgery may not get anxious about the visit. They may have learnt, and are very clear, how to avoid dental treatment. They can therefore successfully manage their dental anxiety. There are more sophisticated observational checklists for systematically noting during short time periods (minimum of a minute) whether a particular behaviour occurs or not (Lee et al. 1989; Melamed & Siegel, 1975). Detailed analysis is possible with observational methods as the treatment sessions can be videotaped and strictly coded using very short time intervals, for example a 4-second duration (Horst & Prins et al. 1987). These methods, however, are time consuming and become very technical. A feature of this method is that the observers must be clear of their definitions when coding. A further consideration is to be aware that the behaviour of the dentist may precipitate a response in the child which may in turn influence the behaviour of the dentist, and so on. Hence simple predictions of child behaviour based on the immediate prior behaviour of the dentist would be inaccurate. In fact it appears that you get an inflated degree of association between the behaviours of the two people unless the previous behaviour of the child was controlled for.

Self-report methods (interviews or questionnaires) have the attraction that the data can be collected relatively quickly. They have great flexibility so that with judicious wording and scoring many different aspects of the dental experience can be rated. However the design of any new questionnaire demands extensive effort and exceptional care at the design stage to enable sense to be made of the data collected. A good example of this is the current use of the Dental Anxiety Scale (DAS) designed by Corah (1969). The scale is short by psychometric standards (see Box 7.6) in that it contains only four questions. However the scale possesses the merit of a high level of internal consistency and some evidence of validity. A modified version (MDAS) has been prepared and used in the UK (Humphris, Morrison & Lindsay 1995). The MDAS is similar to the DAS but includes one additional question about the respondent's feelings to a local anaesthetic injection. The answer scheme has been made consistent across questions. With only five questions the scale can be used routinely in the clinic (see Fig. 7.2). The reliability and validity of the MDAS matches the DAS and in some respects performs more favourably. If used on a regular basis in the dental surgery it gives the clinician:

- An approximate measure of patients' dental anxiety
- Insight into a particular procedure that the patient may be anxious about; and
- Enables comparison of the score to a normative group of patients.

A number of other self-report dental anxiety questionnaires have been designed. Nearly all of them have a larger number of questions than the MDAS which measure other aspects of dental anxiety such as the social consequences of dental

CAN YOU TELL US HOW ANXIOUS YOU GET, IF AT ALL, WITH YOUR DENTAL VISIT ?

PLEASE INDICATE BY INSERTING 'X' IN THE APPROPRIATE BOX

1. If you went to your Dentist for TREATMENT TOMORROW, how would you feel ?

Not Anxious ☐   Slightly Anxious ☐   Fairly Anxious ☐   Very Anxious ☐   Extremely Anxious ☐

2. If you were sitting in the WAITING ROOM (waiting for treatment) how would you feel ?

Not Anxious ☐   Slightly Anxious ☐   Fairly Anxious ☐   Very Anxious ☐   Extremely Anxious ☐

3. If you were about to have a TOOTH DRILLED, how would you feel ?

Not Anxious ☐   Slightly Anxious ☐   Fairly Anxious ☐   Very Anxious ☐   Extremely Anxious ☐

4. If you were about to have your TEETH SCALED AND POLISHED, how would you feel ?

Not Anxious ☐   Slightly Anxious ☐   Fairly Anxious ☐   Very Anxious ☐   Extremely Anxious ☐

5. If you were about to have a LOCAL ANAESTHETIC INJECTION in your gum, above an upper back tooth, how would you feel ?

Not Anxious ☐   Slightly Anxious ☐   Fairly Anxious ☐   Very Anxious ☐   Extremely Anxious ☐

Fig.7.2   The Modified Dental Anxiety Scale (MDAS)

BOX 7.6   PSYCHOMETRICS

Psychometrics is a field of study in which one person is compared with another by providing numerical scores according to that quality the person possesses. A psychometric instrument often consists of a questionnaire with a scoring system that is reliable and valid. Psychometric standards are general criteria that help clinicians decide whether the measure is good for the purposes they wish to use it. Examples of important criteria include:

- The patient can easily comprehend the questionnaire
- It does not tire or upset the patient
- It is reliable (that is, if you were to assess the patient again using the measure you would get virtually the same score)
- It is valid (i.e. it measures what the scale sets out to measure and not other things).

---

anxiety, for example ridicule by friends or family. Even with these scales, however, consisting of numerous questions, some interesting information is still not being assessed.

A helpful distinction to make in measuring anxiety is whether the anxiety is momentary and specific to the situation or whether it is a general response to a wider set of circumstances. These two aspects are referred to as state and trait anxiety. The distinction is important as patients may be very anxious about the dentist but are considered by those who know them socially as being calm and unflustered. This discrepancy may also be distressing to the patient who in other novel situations, even of a medical nature, remains unaffected but may still find the dental situation extremely fearful. It is true however that people may generalise their fear from a specific traumatic occasion, say the snapping of a tooth when an attempt was made to extract it. The resulting surgical operation to remove the embedded root will be unexpected and possibly unpleasant for the patient. The effect of generalisation is shown by the individual becoming anxious the next time he or she approaches the surgery door. The patient may know that the treatment to be conducted is only a simple filling and previously this was not a procedure which caused anxiety.

The importance of pain

A large number of patients expect to experience some pain at the dentist, whereas 11% of patients attending the dentist expect to feel sudden pain at every visit (Lindsay, Humphris & Barnby 1987). It appears a general characteristic that patients tend to expect to feel greater intensity of pain than they actually experience, a finding that has been replicated a number of times with adults and children. What is also interesting is that patients appear to need many visits which are comparatively pain free before reducing their estimate of pain predictions in a future dental visit. This work demonstrates that expectations of pain appear to be fairly stable. An earlier study by Kent (1985) showed that dentally anxious patients rated pain they had experienced as significantly less immediately following treatment compared to their expectation although when they were asked three months later the pain rating had returned to the same as their prediction. This study, replicated by Arntz, has been used to help explain why dental anxiety is resistant to change. If patients are attending on an infrequent basis – say a couple of visits every six months – then this level of positive experience is just not enough to challenge the strongly held beliefs that dental treatment is going to hurt. According to Arntz the anxious patient did not experience greater levels of pain immediately following treatment. What does appear to be important is the maintenance of inaccurate and inflated expectations of pain and the level of anxiety experienced during treatment.

The assessment of pain in these studies has been fairly simplistic, with a heavy reliance on single question assessments. A list of the different assessment methods is presented in Table 7.2. The most popular is the Visual Analogue Scale which is a simple 100 cm line drawn horizontally across the page with the verbal 'anchors' at either end of 'no pain at all' to 'the worst pain imaginable'. The patient is invited to record the pain he experienced (or make his prediction) by placing a short vertical

Table 7.2

Pain assessment methods

Type	Examples	Brief details
Behavioural		
	Facial expression	Criteria based coding of change in facial expression when receiving dental procedure. The eyes, forehead move in a predictable and consistent way which makes a suitable measure.
	Hand grip pressure	Simple technique of child instructed to squeeze a hand grip according to degree of pain intensity experienced.
Self-report		
	Visual Analogue (Scale)	A 100 cm line with 'no pain at all' and (VAS) 'the worst pain imaginable' as descriptors at each end. Patient asked to mark the line to indicate the level of their pain intensity.
	McGill Pain Questionnaire	Sophisticated questionnaire of 20 groups of words which patient selects to show quality of pain experience and can also be converted into an intensity measure of pain.
	Pain Diary	Use of a 1–10 category rating scale of pain intensity to be completed by patient at least daily and sometimes more frequently to show patterns of pain experience over time.

line along the scale. A great deal of effort has been expended to help validate this measure and current opinion tends to recommend that the scale should be divided up into ten segments which helps to avoid 'clumping' of responses. More researchers consider it beneficial to use the more sophisticated McGill Pain Questionnaire which consists of 20 groups of words describing different aspects of pain. The respondent is encouraged to tick which adjective describes their pain most closely. The adjectives are weighted so that a score can be obtained on three separate types of pain which helps to provide a more complex picture of the patient's experience of pain. The three types are listed with examples of how patients may describe their pain in each category:

1. Sensory (e.g. throbbing, shooting, gnawing, aching, smarting)
2. Affective (e.g. exhausting, sickening, frightful, punishing, blinding)
3. Evaluative (e.g. annoying, miserable, unbearable).

When you start to ask your patients about painful sensations, it will be easy to discover more descriptions, to add to this list. The importance of trying to establish what type of pain the patient is describing will give some insight into the response that patients have to their pain experience. For example, those who rate their pain following an extraction as affective in quality such as 'punishing' or 'cruel' will tend to view the dentist in a more negative manner than the patient who describes their pain as 'throbbing' or 'wrenching'.

Pain diaries are less frequently used but may be invaluable in giving a more detailed description over time. Such diaries rely on the patient to steadfastly keep his own record of pain over a period of time, such as days or weeks. The use of these diaries would be appropriate for understanding how a patient might respond to an intervention such as a new painkiller or relaxation procedure to reduce discomfort from tooth extractions or orthodontic treatment. Diaries have been criticised for possibly sensitising patients to their pain. However, some evidence suggests that this effect is small to non-existent when tested with chronic pain patients (Penzien et al. 1994). Pain diaries are especially useful if you want to establish a link between the patient's complaints of pain and some other events that are going on in the patient's life. An example of a pain diary is presented in Chapter 9.

A reliance on self-report methods may be a potential weakness in trying to understand the significance of pain in a patient's response to dentistry and the relationship of pain to anxiety.

This is especially so when attempts are made to directly assess what patients are experiencing at the time of receiving treatment. Other methods have been reported. For example, child patients may be asked to squeeze an airtight rubber bag whenever they feel pain during a dental procedure (Humphris et al. 1991). The degree of squeezing was translated into raising a column of mercury from a sphygmomanometer (used originally for taking blood pressure). This approach was successful in that measures of discomfort can be videotaped and superimposed on a recording of the dental treatment session. Peak and mean levels of pain are retrieved from the recordings. Both measures related strongly to the children's simple five-category VAS rating of experienced pain. This approach allows the experimenter to retrieve pain measures during the dental treatment procedures himself rather than relying on recall.

It is important to be aware that pain is a psychological phenomenon, and does not match the simplistic theory of intensity related to the degree of tissue damage. A number of clear findings have demonstrated that a more complex model of understanding people's experience of pain would be required. The findings may be summarised as follows:

- People experience pain with little or no evidence of organic damage. Patients with atypical facial pain are a clear example from the dental field.
- Patients with extensive physical trauma appear to require very little analgesic and make few complaints about discomfort.
- The placebo effect can produce a measurable change in pain response even though the substance the individual took for the pain was inert. An important influencing factor in achieving a strong effect was for the individual to believe it would reduce their pain. Even if patients are told that the tablet they are taking is a placebo a pain reduction effect may still be achieved.

To account for these effects the Gate Control theory of pain has been proposed. This is regarded as a psychophysiological model, and its main feature is that the information from the sensory nerve receptors is interrupted by a gate in the spinal cord. The function of the gate is to determine the level of the stimulus to transfer from the periphery to the higher centres in the brain which register the stimulus either purely in physical terms, or by generating an emotional response and eventually through connections from the limbic system to the cerebral cortex where the stimulus will be interpreted in the light of previous experience and setting. The Gate Control theory, although elegant and sophisticated enough to account for many pain phenomena, still requires development.

TECHNIQUES OF PAIN REDUCTION

To reduce the pain of dental treatment a number of approaches are available. For example in a recent study to alleviate pain of intraoral injections two approaches were compared with a placebo. The two approaches – topical anaesthesia and transcutaneous electronic nerve stimulation (TENS) – were tested on patients. The topical cream was found to be effective in reducing the pain from palatal injections (using VAS ratings as a measure) compared with the placebo. No effect from the use of TENS was found. TENS is known to be effective for many in the treatment of other forms of pain, such as chronic back pain. The mechanism of action is believed to stimulate sensory nerve fibres in the proximity of the pain location. The stimulation inhibits the perception of pain by 'closing the gate'. The example with local anaesthetic administration, however, was found to be helpful.

There are other ways of reducing treatment pain in the dental context and these approaches may be understood within the framework of the Gate Control theory. One example is the use of audio analgesia. The patient wears headphones through which are passed random frequency sounds (white noise). Clinically, the effect is to distract the patient from the emotive sounds of the treatment. The effect is reliable although it is unlikely to replace more conventional pain relievers.

Individual approach to patient management of dental anxiety

Patients with very high levels of dental anxiety and fear can be helped. A brief introduction to some of the methods that have been experimentally applied in the dental clinic setting are shown below. It is good practice to adopt an individual approach for each patient even though the majority of studies focusing on treating dental anxiety are based upon group comparisons.

TECHNIQUES FOR USE WITH ALL PATIENTS

Counselling and reassurance may be employed almost universally with all patients. Reassurance is not simply saying 'there is no need to worry'. For patients to feel reassured they have to be given information that is fresh and which they can assimilate. A reduction in dental anxiety has been reported in patients who were supplied with an information leaflet at a dental practice. The leaflet was carefully designed to focus on pain control methods for the dentist to adopt and for the patient to be involved in if they wish. For instance, the leaflet contained details of the careful administration of local anaesthetic and the use of stop signals (Jackson & Lindsay 1995).

SPECIFIC TECHNIQUES FOR USE WITH ANXIOUS PATIENTS

Behavioural and cognitive techniques of assisting anxious patients are well known and very successful. It is therefore to be expected that these procedures will perform well to help relieve anxiety in dental patients (Lindsay & Jackson 1993).

Relaxation training

A straightforward procedure widely practised consists of the patient tensing and relaxing various muscle groups in a systematic fashion so that he may appreciate the difference in sensation between tension and release of tension (referred to as tension-release progressive muscular relaxation). The use of tapes and written material to help instruct patients may not be very effective unless the instructor provides feedback to the patient on the success or otherwise of following the relaxation instructions. Applied relaxation, which includes a variety of procedures, may be helpful to focus therapist and patient (Ost 1987). It consists of the following. Firstly, patients keep a detailed record of their anxious feelings (especially physical sensations) so that they become more aware of them. They then learn how to practise the following steps:

- Tension-release progressive relaxation: patients tense up a group of muscles for approximately 20 seconds and then release the tension.
- Release-only relaxation: patients simply attempt to relax a group of muscles.
- Cue-controlled relaxation: this focuses the patient on the words 'inhale' and 'relax' during breathing.
- Differential relaxation: where patients practise their ability to relax in different situations.
- Rapid relaxation: in which patients practise their relaxation skills in more natural surroundings and attempt to quicken the pace of the relaxation process.
- Relaxation under the stresses of the clinic.

Relaxation techniques have been formally tested with dental phobics. For example ten women who self-referred for dental anxiety showed significant improvements following four weeks of cue-controlled relaxation. At six months follow-up eight out of nine of the women found the approach helpful when visiting the dentist (Beck, Kaul & Russell 1978).

Distraction and patient control

Studies to demonstrate the influence of distraction have been conducted in the dental setting. While this is an example of an attempt to enhance control over anxiety symptoms (Kent 1989), this work unfortunately requires replication as it was completed nearly 20 years ago. The distracters employed were simple computer games (table tennis) which may have had novelty value at the time of the study. Measurable effects were however found with dental patients receiving dental treatment in the distraction group showing a significant improvement over the control group. Further work suggests however, that there is a clear preference according to gender – men prefer this method more than women. It would be helpful to ask patients directly what would help them distract their focus from the dental procedure to some harmless and non-distressing mental activity. Note, however, that this approach will not suit everyone. The mental effort of concentrating strongly on another stimulus (imagined or externally generated) can be great and patients may tire easily. This is especially relevant for patients where their main complaint is chronic pain as opposed to fear of dental treatment. Exhortations to try and distract patients from their pain may be helpful for short periods but the psychological strength to maintain a distracting activity for longer periods of time is not realistic.

Patient control of the treatment process (the use of 'stop signals', for example) is a useful and valued procedure well accepted by many patients. Two points should be noted:

- If you do indeed promise to stop on a mutually agreed signal then you *must stop* when indicated by the patient. Failure to do so will damage your relationship.
- Not all patients welcome the opportunity to have that control. Some patients think that this procedure gives the clinician permission to conduct riskier treatment procedures, i.e. you may not be quite so careful and attempt to treat before the local anaesthetic really has had a full chance to work. Alternatively the patient may feel that he has to concentrate more closely on what you are doing and monitor his own somatic sensations more carefully. The heightened arousal required to attend to these stimuli may prevent the patient from adopting his preferred mode of coping such as thinking of pleasant imagery (a coping strategy known as escape-avoidance).

Systematic desensitisation (SD)

> ## Case 7a Patient assisted to confront dental fear gradually
>
> Gender: Male   Age:36   Occupation: Martial arts instructor
>
> Referral: From general dental practitioner (GDP)
>
> Problem: High level of dental anxiety
>
> Features: Patient felt like lashing out at dentist if pain was anticipated
>
> This patient was referred to the joint anxiety clinic at the dental school because of a high level of dental fear. His GDP felt unable to give dental treatment until the patient was less anxious. The patient described his difficulty – the urge to lash out physically against the individual who caused him pain. He had not in fact ever carried out his threat of pushing the clinician away. In a recent visit, however, prior to coming to the dental school he had abruptly left the dental chair while undergoing treatment. It was this event that had prompted his GDP to suggest that he seek some specialist help.
>
> Intervention: He visited one of the authors (GH) for six sessions. These visits focused on his anticipated and distressing outbursts. In addition a behavioural element was included known as systematic desensitisation (SD).

The martial arts instructor was treated psychologically for his high level of dental anxiety by using the approach of systematic desensitisation. The SD procedure consisted of obtaining, through talking with the patient, a hierarchy of fears, teaching a relaxation technique and gradually exposing the patient to each stage of his fear hierarchy starting with sitting in the dental chair.

This case is typical of a dentally anxious patient trying to come to terms with his intensely uncomfortable feelings about a visit to the dentist.

Discussion focused on the patient's possible loss of control during the desensitisation exercises. The gradual exposure to each stage of his fear hierarchy enabled him to inspect at first hand his experience of wanting to leave the surgery. This desire to leave is an example of trying to avoid further exposure to the patient's feared objects (the syringe and the drill). He admitted to being very ashamed and embarrassed by his phobia. He became convinced that his threat of causing the clinician some unintended harm was a way for him to retain the strong and unflinching image which he typically presented to his martial art students. It was explained to him that his desire to leave the situation was to be expected – however the way to reduce avoidance was by repeated visits to the surgery. This approach behaviour would make him more familiar (a process known as habituation) with the experience of wanting to leave. In encouraging him to visit frequently, he was able to recognise that it would improve his ability to tolerate the strong urge to leave. It was explained to him that (i) his difficulty was a natural reaction, and one of which the dental team was aware; and (ii) that his treatment would be halted immediately and he would be allowed to leave the surgery if necessary. These procedures provided a means for the patient to accept treatment consisting of a number of restorations with local anaesthetic injections.

This case demonstrates a way of assisting the patient to confront situations he was afraid of, and presenting a suitable framework to help him accept a view of himself as a potent and physically fit man who had the ability to deal with extreme provocation in a calm and considered manner. He was encouraged to think that his difficulty required some extra attention on his part to recognise that his fear could be managed with some gradual but persistent effort. The embarrassment of not being able to receive dental treatment was considerable and this element required sensitive attention to prevent him taking offence. Two principles are demonstrated with this case, namely confrontation or exposure to the thing (e.g. the drill) that causes fear and assistance in thinking differently and more positively about the individual's response to feared objects. In summary this case illustrates:

- You may meet anxious patients in the surgery who do not fit your expected (stereotypical) view.
- The patient's reaction to dentistry is very often linked to the social context from which he comes (or as in this case the patient's occupation).
- The anxious feelings patients experience make them want to leave the surgery as quickly as possible.
- The patient will readily accept excuses to avoid treatment.
- Exposing patients to their fears in a structured and considerate manner is helpful.
- Patients are often embarrassed by their fears.

Systematic desensitisation (SD) treatment includes a number of specific steps.

- The compilation of a fear hierarchy, in which the patient is encouraged to state the aspects of dental experience of which he is afraid, and then to place them in a rank order of fear, starting with the least fearful and progressing to the most fearful (1–2 sessions).
- The patient is taught relaxation procedures (2–3 sessions).
- Finally the patient approaches the situation that is the lowest stage of fear in his hierarchy. Once the patient is able to tolerate that stage then encouragement is given to proceed to the next. The hierarchy is an important negotiation process with patients and can provide useful information about the fears they hold (five or more sessions depending on progress and length of hierarchy).

In a well-designed study comparing the effects of systematic desensitisation with general anaesthesia (GA) on dental phobics Berggren found that the dental anxiety (assessed by the DAS) of those patients treated with SD was significantly less than those given GA. In addition the most important finding was that the relapse rate for dental anxiety was considerably less for the SD compared to the GA group. The reasons for discontinuing treatment were significantly more numerous in the GA group than the SD group. The decline of dental anxiety was still measurable at ten-year follow-up (Hakeburg, Berggren & Carlsson 1990).

Case 7b   A special case of severe dental anxiety

Gender: Female   Age: 25   Occupation: Unemployed
Referral: From pedodontic unit, dental hospital
Problem: Severe dental anxiety, approaching phobia
Features: Experiencing dental pain from suspected abscess, traumatic experience at six years of age, serious sexual assault at 20 years of age

A referral was received from the pedodontic unit within the dental school, where the patient had been treated intermittently up to a couple of years ago. She had received relative analgesia in her patchy visits to the unit but treatment had always remained a difficulty. After an absence of two years she returned requesting treatment as she was getting some pain from one of her teeth and she suspected an abscess was forming. She was very nervous on examination in the dental surgery and hence was referred to a clinical psychologist. In the first session the patient explained that although she was appreciative of the help she had received from the children's unit she was aware that she needed to be treated in the adult services, and had become self-conscious of waiting with young children before being seen. She had had a negative experience of a dental appointment at the age of six when she attended for an extraction. She explained that she was receiving psychotherapy for depression and took antidepressants and mild tranquilisers when required. She recounted a traumatic sexual assault some five years ago which had caused her depression. The male assailant had locked her in the house to prevent her escape from an ordeal which lasted some hours.

Where it is difficult to expose the patient directly to the dental situation, for example when patients are seen initially in a consulting room or office, it may be appropriate to instruct patients to practise 'imaginal' SD. That is the patient is encouraged to imagine that she is entering a dental surgery, is able to sit in the dental chair and eventually able to receive dental treatment. This approach will strengthen the capacity of the individual to believe that she can complete the programme in a real-life setting when she enters the surgery.

Such an approach was adopted with this woman who had been subjected to a particularly violent attack in her own home. The circumstances of the assault were important details in the explanation of her difficulty in receiving dental treatment, and in suggesting how her anxiety could be managed. This and further information was given by the patient in a single session demonstrating that patients are sometimes ready to divulge sensitive information when they are aware that it will be listened to sympathetically and would encourage a clearer response to treatment. In addition the fact that this patient had already had extensive psychotherapy enabled her to relate her traumatic experience. Three components of treatment were applied:

1. Imaginal desensitisation (ID) was conducted as the patient did not feel able to enter a dental surgery with a dentist present without some form of preparation. A small number of sessions were required for her to imagine being successful in attending the dentist and having an examination. While she was imagining these events, she was encouraged to remain as relaxed as possible. If she felt anxious she was instructed to stop the scenario running in her mind and discuss what she felt.

2. Only when she felt comfortable about rehearsing the examination in her mind was she encouraged to attempt actual visits to the dentist in a gradual manner, while still keeping relaxed (that is, systematic desensitisation).

3. Another component of the psychological intervention consisted of providing the patient with a detailed map of the building and repeated tours of the entrance/exit, corridors, stairwells and clinic areas. The patient expressed great apprehension about getting lost and not being able to leave the dental school. Therefore it was stressed to the patient that she could leave the dental chair whenever

she wished, and if necessary the building. This was rehearsed with the patient on a number of occasions.

The patient was offered an appointment with a female dentist which she accepted. A 'handover' session was organised so that the psychologist introduced the patient to the dentist and the aspects of treatment which caused her difficulty were reiterated. The dentist explained the procedures and reminded the patient that she could leave the surgery and the premises whenever she wished. The surgery door was left wide open to support this approach. The patient responded well and required about three treatment sessions in which she received some restorations. The case demonstrates that the embarrassment and shame that patients feel when they suffer extreme levels of anxiety can be severe and the result of a number of experiences not always linked to traumatic dental episodes. The effect of previous trauma and associations with elevated dental fear has been supported by a survey conducted in Seattle, USA (Walker et al. 1996). The authors found that high dental fear among women was significantly associated with a higher prevalence of several forms of childhood maltreatment and adult sexual and physical abuse. Hence some patients will come for dental treatment with substantial psychological problems in addition to their difficulties in accepting treatment. It should be noted that these comments do not infer traumatic experiences are necessarily responsible for dental anxieties, but rather that you should be alert to a wider range of factors that may be implicated in the care of dental patients. In Chapters 8 and 9 there is further discussion of the social and psychological factors associated with a number of dental conditions.

General comments on dental anxiety

It is important to treat the patient as an individual. In order to do this some detailed assessment is required which will use some of the questionnaires referred to already. In addition the dentist will need to employ some of the communication skills outlined in Chapter 6 to encourage the patient to relate the nature of his or her difficulty. Patients may be distressed or embarrassed and need reassurance.

Methods of assisting dentally anxious patients that require minimal intervention are advocated, especially with the current emphasis on value-for-money services. New patients have been shown how to reduce their dental anxiety by being given an information leaflet which focuses on pain control and the use of stop signals, as mentioned previously. What is interesting with this approach is that the authors compared their leaflet with one which simply expressed sympathy with the patient's distress. This suggests that expressions of sympathy alone are probably not sufficient to reduce dental anxiety.

A clinical trial designed to assess the influence of a single session of cognitive treatment of dental phobia found substantial short-term improvements in reducing negative thinking (cognitions) and dental anxiety in both frequency and believability, when compared to waiting list controls and a patient receiving information about oral health and dental treatment. Both interventions lasted one hour. The difference between the information and cognitive restructuring (see Box 7.7) was not confirmed at one-year follow-up which tends to show that some extra involvement in the cognitive approach may be required on a more frequent basis to maintain superiority over simply supplying information (de Jongh et al. 1995a). Minimal interventions may be valuable for those with moderate anxiety levels which prevent patients from making their regular dental appointments. A four-session clinical trial with anxious students was conducted that consisted of an intensive approach using desensitisation and giving students live feedback of their galvanic skin response (see Box 7.5). The biofeedback-assisted desensitisation was consistently effective (Denney, Rupert & Burish 1983). An important factor for success in helping patients is to ensure that they gain experience of managing their anxiety response themselves as opposed to simply being provided with an educational/informational package (Moses & Hollandsworth 1985).

BOX 7.7   COGNITIVE RESTRUCTURING

This is an approach in which the clinician encourages patients to think differently about the situations that they find threatening. Specifically patients are asked to look at the evidence on which they base their beliefs and to question how well they can rely on the underlying beliefs that they hold. It is a method which attempts to change patients' views in order to become more realistic about their fears and the situations that can cause them. The approach has to be applied with some care in order not to cause offence but to gently invite patients to inspect their reasons for holding unrealistic fears. This is done for example by conducting mini-experiments: for example, encouraging the patient to make an appointment with a dentist purely to discuss treatment and determine, following the appointment, that the patient's catastrophic thoughts that the dentist would launch into invasive treatment at the first session were incorrect.

STABILITY OF DENTAL ANXIETY

Although there is a formidable set of techniques which may be used – simple varieties of relaxation, patients controlling the pace of treatment and systematic desensitisation – there are likely to be patients with dental anxiety who do not improve. Reasons for the lack of reduction in anxiety may not necessarily be because of the inefficiency of the technique or the lack of skill of the clinician (see however Box 7.8). It is likely that the factors maintaining the high level of dental anxiety should be given greater attention by the clinician through further assessment. Reasons for anxiety remaining stable are listed in Table 7.3. It may be that at this stage the patient requires more specialist help. The general medical practitioner should be informed, with the patient, to encourage a referral to the local clinical psychology service. Alternatively a list of clinical psychologists in the UK is now available (the Directory of Chartered Psychologists) in reference libraries.

Table 7.3

Theoretical explanations for dental anxiety remaining stable

Theoretical 'family'	Explanation
Learning theory	Too few exposure episodes (i.e. dental visits) for habituation to dental stimuli.
	Too short an exposure time (i.e. typical treatment episode may last for 20 minutes). Optimum time for exposure is approximately 45 minutes.
Cognitive theory	Less frequency of painful experiences due to improved local anaesthetic procedures will increase concern that a painful experience is more likely on the next visit. In addition more visits will be necessary before the patient can believe that pain is very unlikely.
	Exposure to feared stimuli (e.g. needles, syringes) in an SD programme may not reduce fear if patients regard the experience as untypical (clinicians therefore need to design their programmes to mimic closely the experience that the patient will have when undergoing treatment). Situational factors should be matched if at all possible, i.e. conduct sessions in the dental surgery that the patient will receive actual treatment.

BOX 7.8   WHEN ANXIETY LEVELS DO NOT REDUCE

Some reasons for systematic desensitisation not being effective:

- The fear hierarchy is not specific to the fear expressed by the patient (for example, a patient who is fearful of the needle being injected into the gum as opposed to the clinician's hierarchy that encourages the patient to be comfortable about seeing needles).
- The clinician may be going too fast and not enabling the patient to make sense of changed responses to previously fear-provoking images or actions.

- The hierarchy may not be graded finely enough.
- Appointments are too widely spaced apart or too brief.

Some reasons for cognitive restructuring not being effective:

- Premature use of the technique before the assumptions used by the patient have been properly discovered.
- Patient not prepared properly in understanding the joint endeavour.
- Patients unable to present their thoughts or finding it too distressing or ridiculous.
- The clinician does most of the 'work' for the patient, and the patient feels uninvolved.

Dental anxiety in children

Estimates of dental fear in children are more difficult to collect and interpret than in adults. Some self-report questionnaires are available (see Box 7.9). Parental reports, although useful, are likely to be biased, either to present their child favourably or include a reflection of their own anxiety which the child tends not to share. Observations of children attending for dental treatment provide an objective attempt at measurement (Aartman et al. 1996), although even children who receive dental treatment may still be very afraid. A US survey found that, five per cent of children were unable to receive all of their treatment when attending the dentist. A large study in Sweden found that 79% of children aged 3–16 years attending the dentist positively accepted all dental treatment, 13% reluctantly accepted and 8% presented a negative reaction or did not accept treatment. A dentist training programme introduced the intervention of behaviour shaping (also known as tell-show-do, with an emphasis on positive reinforcement). The corresponding figures for acceptance after the training were 92%, 6% and 2%. The improvement was clearest among the younger children and those

requiring restorative treatment or extraction. The authors found that treatment time was not extended using this intervention (Holst & Ek 1988).

BOX 7.9   ASSESSMENT OF DENTAL ANXIETY IN CHILDREN

If you wish to measure children's dental anxiety in a systematic way then consider using the following questionnaires. All of them are completed by the children themselves. The clinician may need to read the questions through with the child, but without giving a prompt. Even with reading the questions, very young children are best excluded from using these scales, with the exception of the Venham scale which is easy to answer.

Name of scale	Length (no. of questions)	Comments
Children's Dental Fear Survey Schedule	15	The most comprehensive scale. Extensively used. International norms available. Fairly long. Good reliability and validity.
Corah's Dental Anxiety Scale (child version)	4	Short. Familiar because of adult scale. It has similar problems to the adult scale, however, as the answering categories are a little confusing. There is no question about needles/injections.
Venham's Scale	8	This comprises eight pairs of cartoon figures of children in various states of anxiety. Child has to select which picture of the pair he or she regards as most like themselves. Simple scoring method. Suitable for children as young as three years of age. Measures 'state' dental anxiety.
Modified Child Dental Anxiety Scale	8	Similar to the Corah DAS, but extended and with simplified method for child to answer. Useful for trials to test new interventions. UK norms only.

Many of the procedures that have been presented with adults may be adapted for use with children, although developmental level is an important additional factor. Young children will interpret certain sensations and instructions differently – for example, pain felt as a result of some dental procedure may be interpreted with some magical or perhaps sinister qualities. The feeling of being reprimanded or punished when visiting the dentist for some invasive dental treatment is common and the clinician must encourage the child to believe that he has coped well with the experience. Positive reinforcement (i.e. 'behaviour shaping') at every stage of the treatment process is recommended, to indicate to the child that he is making successful steps in the process of receiving treatment. The frequent use of praise during a child's appointment – when the child performs an appropriate behaviour – is essential. The dialogue below provides an example.

Dentist:	Let's have a look inside your mouth. Please open your mouth as wide as you can.
Child patient:	[Opens mouth slightly but not enough to allow dentist to complete examination].
Dentist:	You are starting to open you mouth lovely and wide so that I can begin to see your teeth. Show me now how well you can open your mouth.
Child patient:	[Opens mouth wider at request so that dentist can start to look at child's teeth].
Dentist:	You have opened your mouth really well. I am pleased with how well you can open your mouth.

Note that you need to reward the child with praise at each stage to encourage the behaviour you wish the child to present. This will be more successful than providing a single large reinforcement (for example, a badge, leaflet or tube of toothpaste) at the end of the examination. This is an example of *operant conditioning*, where the positive reinforcement of a specific behaviour such as mouth opening will encourage the child to continue and make the chance of that behaviour more likely in the future. Equally, you should ignore mildly disruptive behaviour as this will become less frequent if the child does not receive reinforcement to continue with it. Sometimes behaviour cannot be ignored – such as the child who tries to clutch the

syringe just prior to an injection. This potentially dangerous behaviour has to be prevented and cannot be ignored. A firmly worded instruction can be given to the child. However you should encourage the child by explaining exactly what you would like him to do and giving praise in stages when he behaves close to the required level that will allow you to complete the procedure. Frequent and well-delivered praise can achieve excellent results in encouraging children to receive dental treatment.

MODELLING

Melamed and Siegel (1975) have reported a number of key studies illustrating the positive effects that watching a video of other children undergoing procedures similar to the ones they will undergo can have on dentally naïve and anxious children. Especially successful models are those with children who express some difficulty in receiving dental treatment – they say on film that they are nervous – but are shown to be able to master their fear and successfully receive the treatment.

VOICE CONTROL

Moderating the pitch and volume of the voice has been experimentally tested with child dental patients. Using a moderately raised voice has been shown to improve adherence to dental procedures and result in less complaining behaviour.

USE OF PHARMACOLOGICAL ASSISTANCE IN CHILDREN

A randomised double-blind study investigating the effectiveness of nitrous oxide on disruptive behaviour and successfully received dental treatment was conducted by Weinstein, Domoto & Holleman (1986). In the only study of its kind (that is, a double-blind clinical trial) it was found that there were no significant differences between the experimental nitrous oxide and control air groups. The influence of the dentist interacting with the nitrous oxide intervention, however, showed a positive effect. This study was remarkable for its attention to detail in the design, and the assiduousness of the behavioural ratings (all videotaped and coded using a validated system of classification of the child's behaviour through the treatment period). It demonstrated that the use of pharmacological aids such as nitrous oxide required the dentist to assist in calming the child in order to allow treatment to progress.

Conclusion

The strategies for managing patient fears and anxieties from a psychological perspective are varied and careful assessment is required to match the management strategy to the patients' difficulties. An openness with patients characterises the nature in which many of these interventions have been developed. There is now a need to study the success of fitting the intervention to the particular distress of the patient. In general the strategies described above work well especially with people who have discrete specific problems of dental anxiety and fear. When patients have additional problems such as depression, panic attacks, agoraphobia or obsessions for example, then the relatively focused approaches listed in this chapter may be insufficient (see Chapter 9).

References

Aartman I, van Everdingen T, Hoogstraten J, Schuurs A 1996 Appraisal of behavioural measurement techniques for assessing dental anxiety and fear in children: A review. Journal of Psychopathology and Behavioral Assessment 18(2):153–171

Beck F, Kaul T, Russell R 1978 Treatment of dental anxiety by cue-controlled relaxation. Journal of Counselling Psychology 25(6):591–594

Conway M 1995 Flashbulb Memories. Hove, UK: Lawrence Erlbaum Associates

Corah N L 1969 Development of a dental anxiety scale. Journal of Dental Research 48:596

Davey G C L 1989 Dental phobias and anxieties: evidence for conditioning processes in the acquisition and modulation of a learned fear. Behaviour Research and Therapy 27(1):51–58

de Jongh A, Muris P, ter Horst G, van Zuuren F 1995a. One-session cognitive treatment of dental phobia: preparing dental phobics for treatment by restructuring negative cognitions. Behaviour Research and Therapy 33(8):947–954

de Jongh A, ter Horst G, Muris P, Merckerlbach H 1995b. Looking at threat-relevant stimuli: The role of anxiety and coping style. Anxiety, Stress and Coping 8(1):37–45

Denney D, Rupert P, Burish T 1983. Skin conductance biofeedback and desensitisation for reducing dental anxiety. American Journal of Clinical Biofeedback, 6(2):88–95

Frankl S N, Shiere F R, Fogels H R 1962 Should the parent remain with the child in the dental operatory? Journal of Dentistry for Children, 29:150–163

Freeman R 1998 A psychodynamic theory of dental phobia. British Dental Journal 184:170–172

Hakeburg M, Berggren U, Carlsson S G 1990 A 10-year follow-up of patients treated for dental fear. Scandinavian Journal of Dental Research 98:53–59

Holst A, Ek L 1988 Effect of systematized 'behavior shaping' on acceptance of dental treatment in children. Community Dentistry and Oral Epidemiology 16:349–355

Humphris G M, Mair L, Lee G T R, Birch R H 1991 Dental anxiety, pain and uncooperative behaviour in child dental patients. Anxiety Research 4:61–77

Humphris G M, Morrison T, Lindsay S J E 1995 The Modified Dental Anxiety Scale: UK norms and evidence for validity. Community Dental Health 12: 143–150

Jackson C, Lindsay S 1995 Reducing anxiety in new dental patients by means of leaflets. British Dental Journal 179:163–167

Kent G 1985 Memory of dental pain. Pain 21:187–194

Kent G 1989 Cognitive aspects of the maintenance and treatment of dental anxiety: a review. Journal of Cognitive Psychotherapy 3(3):201–221

Kent G, Croucher R (eds.) 1998 Achieving oral health (3rd edn.) London: Wright

Lee G T R, Humphris G M, Birch R H, Mair L 1989 Disruptive behaviour during dental treatment of uncooperative children. Journal of Pediatric Dentistry 14:27–30

Lindsay S J E, Humphris G M, Barnby G J 1987 Expectations and preferences for routine dentistry in anxious adult patients. British Dental Journal 163:120–124

Lindsay S J E, Jackson C 1993 Fear of routine dental treatment in adults: its nature and management. Psychology and Health 8(2,3):165–174

Melamed B G, Siegel L J 1975 Reduction of anxiety of children facing hospitalisation and surgery by use of filmed modelling. Journal of Consulting and Clinical Psychology 43(4):511–521

Moore R, Brodsgard I, Birn H 1991. Manifestations, acquisition and diagnostic categories of dental fear in a self-referred population. Behaviour Research and Therapy 29:51–60

Moses A, Hollandsworth J 1985. Relative effectiveness of education alone versus stress inoculation training in the treatment of dental phobia. Behaviour Therapy 16(5):531–537

Murray P, Liddell A, Donohue J 1989 A longitudinal study of the contribution of dental experiences to dental anxiety in children between 9 and 12 years of age. Journal of Behavioral Medicine 12(3):309–320

Ost L G 1987 Applied relaxation: description of a coping technique and a review of controlled studies. Behaviour Research and Therapy 25:397–410

Penzien D B, Johnson C A, Seville J L, Rubman S, Boggess J T, Rains J C 1994 Interrelationships among daily and global self-report measures of headache. Headache Quarterly–Current Treatment Research 5:27–33 ter Horst G, Prins P J M, et al. 1987 Interactions between dentists and anxious child patients: a behavioural analysis. Community Dentistry and Oral Epidemiology, 15:249–252

ter Horst G, de Wit C A 1993 Review of behavioural research in dentistry 1987–1992: dental anxiety, dentist–patient relationship, compliance and dental attendance. International Dental Journal 43:265–278

Todd J E, Lader D 1991 Adult dental health: 1988. United Kingdom OPCS Survey Division. London: HMSO

Vassend O 1993 Anxiety, pain and discomfort associated with dental treatment. Behaviour Research and Therapy 31(7):659–666

Vignehsa H, Chellappah N K, Milgrom P et al. 1990. A clinical evaluation of high- and low-fear children in Singapore. Journal of Dentistry for Children 57:224–228

Walker E A, Milgrom P M, Weinstein P, Getz T, Richardson R 1996 Assessing abuse and neglect and dental fear in women. Journal of the American Dental Association 127:485–490

Weinstein P, Domoto P, Holleman E 1986 The use of nitrous oxide in the treatment of children: results of a controlled study. Journal of the American Dental Association 112:325–321

PART 3

PSYCHOSOCIAL FACTORS AND ORAL HEALTH

8

Psychosocial factors in the aetiology of oral health problems

This chapter explores aspects of psychosocial factors which are a contributory cause of oral health problems. Four examples are presented, and each is illustrated by a case. It can be argued that there are many instances where social and psychological factors influence oral health. The first two cases have been chosen to show how these factors could cause instances of caries and periodontal disease. Our understanding is incomplete. However, it is important for the clinician to be aware of ways in which oral health can be compromised: it is possible that you can prevent such problems by attempting to change these causative factors – for example, by using persuasion to alter individual health beliefs (Case 8a) or advising patients to consider adapting their lifestyle (Case 8b).

Case 8a   Parental health beliefs and a child's dental health

A health visitor, making a postnatal visit to a family with a three-week-old baby boy and a two-year-old girl noticed that the mother, when preparing a drink for the girl gave her a fruit cordial which although diluted with water had a high sugar content.

The health visitor was rather surprised by this behaviour, especially as the mother was a schoolteacher who was at the time on maternity leave. During conversation the mother mentioned that the baby was already taking plain boiled water between his feeds – she explained how she had adopted a similar practice with her elder child. She had subsequently introduced the sugary drink

---

because her daughter would not eat fruit, and she felt that the benefits of the vitamin C in the drink outweighed the disadvantages of the drink's high sugar content, especially as her daughter had good oral hygiene. She concluded by emphasising that her action was further justified because deciduous teeth were less important than permanent teeth. The health visitor responded to this by explaining the risks to permanent dentition by caries in deciduous teeth. She then discussed with the mother alternative ways of addressing her concern that her daughter's diet could be deficient in vitamin C.

This case was observed by one of the authors during fieldwork involving a study concerning the work of health visitors, and focuses on:

- Preventive approaches
- The benefit of using the skills of different members of the primary healthcare team when providing preventive advice to individuals
- The socialisation of children.

Informal or primary socialisation permits the norms and values of the mother to be passed on to the child, particularly with regard to dietary habits. Mothers are thus regarded as key figures in dental health (Blinkhorn 1989; Grytten et al. 1988; Kay & McGuiness 1990).

Graham (1985) emphasises a different aspect of the role of the mother, stating that the wife-mother as principal carer, acts as a gatekeeper between the family and the outside world. She decides about the utilisation of lay and professional services.

One example of this is the way in which many mothers act to directly control, or at least heavily influence, their children's oral health. This occurs both by their influence on oral hygiene practices, including the use of dental services, and through the effects of the food and drink they provide for their children and encourage or discourage them to consume.

Complexity of lay beliefs

An important issue raised by this case concerns the complexity associated with the mother's beliefs about oral health and disease, particularly regarding sugar consumption. The mother explained carefully to the health visitor the rationale underlying her action, conveying that she understood the importance of actively promoting good oral health. This she achieved by giving plain boiled water rather than sugary drinks to her children when babies. She explained how in her role as a teacher she had worked very hard to discourage the sale of sugary foods at break times. This was done because of her awareness of the cariogenic nature of sugar and its destructive role in the pupils' oral health.

However, in the case of her own two-year-old daughter, concern for what she regarded as a deficiency in the child's diet caused her to adapt her practice regarding the drinks she provided.

PUBLIC AND PRIVATE ACCOUNTS

A study by Backett (1990) showed similar forms of adaptation regarding adherence to ideals of healthy living. Backett used in-depth interviews which took place four times over an 18 month period to explore the health beliefs and attitudes of families in Edinburgh. The families comprised married couples and dependent children – family structures similar to Case 8a. From this work Backett suggested that there existed three distinct accounts about health beliefs and attitudes.

1. Predominantly 'public' accounts which reflect respondents' perceptions of social norms and morally approved codes of behaviour.

2. Generalised accounts of what 'usually happens'.
3. Some participants offered 'private' accounts (for example by personal anecdote).

In Case 8a the health visitor, who had visited this particular family several times, received a mixture of these different types of account (Backett 1990).

Interpreting situations

The focus on private and public accounts illustrates the need to interpret the accounts and explanations given by patients. It is also important to have regard for how well the professional knows the patient and the extent to which the clinician has previously discussed the issue concerned. Blinkhorn, in a discussion of preventive dental regimens based in the dental surgery, advocated spending time not only on dietary counselling, but also of offering regular reinforcement of advice (Blinkhorn 1993). He also remarked on the need not to be disillusioned if changes in behaviour are not instantly successful.

Effecting changes in attitudes or behaviour requires the professional to achieve a sufficient understanding of the patient's/client's situation for the advice offered to be both appropriate and accepted. The health visitor involved in this case considered that she was in a particularly favourable position because she was able to visit individuals in their own homes. Visiting clients' homes, rather than their having to go to the professional, was seen by the health visitor as a means of 'closing the gap' between herself and her clients. A home visit often enabled her to broach difficult issues, such as that of the sugary drink, because she had observed the situation at first hand. However, she also commented upon how careful she had to be during home visits not to appear as an 'interfering busybody' (Symmonds 1991).

CONFLICTING CONCERNS

A further issue to be raised from listening to patients carefully is that a patient's actions are usually influenced by a variety of often conflicting concerns and are typically based on an incomplete knowledge or understanding. In such situations their decisions and behaviour are strongly influenced by what they perceive as socially acceptable practice and as commonsense. Indeed, the explanations or accounts that they give to professionals may often be based on what they feel constitutes an acceptable justification for their action. In some ways this explanatory framework is similar to the more formal models presented in Chapter 10 which focus on the way in which beliefs, attitudes and social pressures may influence dental health behaviour.

In Case 8a however, the woman's rationalisation of her daughter's deciduous teeth being temporary may be interpreted as a form of defence. By contrast the issue of her daughter's diet and the high vitamin C content of the drink should be seen as the positive reason offered for her behaviour. The mother appears to have been acting from wholly well-intended motives and with a genuine concern for maintaining good health for her daughter. Her behaviour, although incorrect, would seem to have arisen from her lack of understanding regarding the relationship between the health of deciduous and permanent dentition.

CONTRADICTORY CONCERNS

In other situations, people may behave in ways that they know cause harm to health, but where they believe such harm is outweighed by other benefits, perhaps unrelated to health. Such tradeoffs often arise in situations where lack of resources, whether financial or time, preclude the person from behaving in a way that would enable them to achieve the benefits they seek without risking harm to health.

Although discussing 'the conflicts that go with caring for health in circumstances of hardship', Graham (1993) describes how 'a very contradictory kind of support' is used by some mothers regarding the place of sweets in the lives of their children. These mothers give their children sweets. Such sweets are an affordable way of permitting their children's lifestyles to match those of their peers. In this situation the mothers would seem to regard sacrificing the child's dental health as worthwhile to gain a mixture of social inclusion for the child and avoidance of social stigma for the family. It

may also represent an easy way for the parents to respond to at least some of the demands made by their children and so avoid conflict within the family. Therefore, mothers may well cope in ways which promote family welfare, in the encouragement of good relationships between parents and children but which undermines individual health. This example provides an illustration of the complexities which are often faced by healthcare professionals when providing preventive advice to patients. Having considered, by exploration of this case, aspects of prevention and aetiology, the next two cases will discuss the psychosocial factors of the aetiology associated with existing oral health problems.

Case 8b   Can stress influence dental health?

Gender: Male   Age: 32   Occupation:
                                            Sales executive
Referral: Self-referral to local general dental practice
Problem: Complains of ulcers suddenly appearing on the gums
Features: Under pressure from work and difficult home life

This patient called in to his dentist to ask for advice, complaining of ulcers along the gum line. His wife had insisted that he come to the dentist as she had noticed that his breath smelt dreadful. The patient had been reluctant at first, as he was so busy keeping up with his work schedule, but to avoid further disagreement with his wife he decided he should seek some help. On examination his dentist said that his periodontal condition was not particularly good and that he was suffering from acute ulcerative gingivitis. Topical antibiotic gel and an antiseptic mouthwash were prescribed. As the patient was a long-standing friend of the dentist – they had both been to the same school – the patient confided that he was under a great deal of stress, and had been to his doctor to complain of a dry mouth and headaches. The doctor had suggested that he was suffering from general that he was suffering from general anxiety, which was causing his tension headaches and reducing his salivary flow. It was clear that as well as major organisational changes being introduced at his workplace there were some problems with his marriage. The patient was not able to go into detail except to say that the bringing up of his two young sons (two and four years of age) had introduced substantial pressures into the household. The mother had recently returned to full-time work and he had not realised that he needed to be more flexible in his own work arrangements to allow both parents to meet their home and work responsibilities.

This case is interesting as it shows that there may be a very close correspondence between an individual's lifestyle and the incidence of oral disease. Whereas the previous case (8a) demonstrated a complex set of factors which led to a deterioration in the child's primary dentition, the influence on dental health was more long standing. Caries takes time to develop and the cause of this form of dental disease is truly multifactorial (i.e. many aspects of the child's life were effective in producing the conditions for caries to develop). The sales executive however suffered from an acute disease which seemed to be linked to his marital problems.

Changes in our lives can result in positive or negative effects. Where there is extensive change requiring many adjustments then individuals report them as being stressful. This can be true even with many positive events (e.g. following a jackpot win on the lottery). When these events are unpredictable or uncontrollable then increases in stress are perceived. A scale has been developed by Holmes and Rahe (1967) to measure the level of life events that an individual has experienced over, say, a period of a year (Box 8.1). Each life event was rated by a large sample of people and assigned a value to indicate the degree of readjustment required. A greater impact was made with negative rather than positive events. To calculate the life event score, all the events that have occurred over the past 12 months are listed for the individual and simply summed to give a score. The higher the score on the scale, the greater the amount of

adjustment is required. If this level of life events continues for a lengthy period then the greater the likelihood of chronic stress. It is important to note that there are large variations in the response to these events. Some students for example find exams a chance to learn about their strengths as opposed to focusing on the possibility of failure.

There is substantial indirect evidence that physiological mechanisms are interrupted or disturbed by events in people's lives. Continued adjustments to prolonged stressors may weaken the body's resources. An event experienced as a stressor may activate the hypothalamus which operates the sympathetic nervous system. This system sends out nervous impulses that directly affect internal organs and glands. For instance the salivary glands are inhibited by the sympathetic nervous activity and salivary flow is reduced – the periodontal tissue is more prone to infection without the presence of saliva.

BOX 8.1 LIFE EVENTS SCALE	
Life event	Value
Death of spouse	100
Divorce	73
Marital separation	65
Prison sentence	63
Death of close family member	63
Personal injury or illness	53
Marriage	50
Pregnancy	40
Death of close friend	37
Change in responsibilities at work	29
Son or daughter leaving home	29
Starting or leaving school	26
Change in residence	20
Change in social activities	18
Holiday	13
Christmas	12
(Example items from the Holmes and Rahe scale, with values used to assess extent of perceived stress)	

The immune system is believed to be responsive to the levels of stress to which people are exposed. Human immune functioning is a complex system and there are many approaches to assessing its competence. The greater the level of stress the less efficient the immune system is in protecting the individual from disease and infection. For instance, research has shown that men and women who have experienced a divorce or separation show reduced immune functioning when compared with people who are still married. Further work has shown that the immune function, as recorded by a number of indices (such as lymphocyte count), improves when people regularly practise relaxation training. These results suggest that the ability of individuals to withstand microbial infection is reduced during periods of intense pressure.

In a large sample of civil servants (over 3000) a study investigated whether eight specific life events were associated with oral symptoms. These symptoms were reported by the civil servants themselves rather than by oral examination, and self-report methods enabled questions to be asked about these symptoms over the past year (chronic) and in the last 14 days (acute). A number of life events were found to be related either to acute or chronic oral symptoms. The life events implicated included marital or family problems, bereavement, personal serious illness, the serious illness of a close relative, major financial difficulty, mugging and robbery. The list of events that are related to oral symptoms are similar to the original stressful life event list presented by Holmes and Rahe.

A different and less direct route is through oral health behaviour itself. For instance, the patient in Case 8b may have had less time to devote to oral hygiene practices in the last few weeks, or his diet may have been impoverished by rushing to meet deadlines and obligations. He may have ingested sugar-containing foods and drinks more frequently because of his hurried schedule. A dry mouth may have encouraged him to eat sucrose sweets to stimulate more saliva, or to act as a psychological comfort to induce relaxation. What is important to appreciate is that the way people lead their lives (referred to as lifestyle factors) or what life events they have been exposed to, may help to explain, to some extent, their oral symptoms. The manner in which this effect can occur is through a person's stress response.

The skills of professional helpers, be they dental personnel or nurses, in assisting people with

Case 8c Facial appearance and depression

Gender: Female   Age: 66   Occupation: Retired beauty therapist
Referral: Secondary referral from prosthetics consultant
Problem: Concern over appearance
Features: Depressed from increased social isolation

This patient was keen to receive implants: she was very distressed with her own dentures which clearly were poorly fitting. It was noticeable that her lower denture was displaced at an angle and her upper denture on occasion fell when her mouth opened. From an initial brief discussion it emerged that she was so concerned about her appearance that she felt unable to go out. This in turn was making her feel isolated and depressed. She indicated that she was near the end of her tether. On asking her what she meant by this, she stated that she would never take her own life but that she did feel desperate.

Two interview sessions were planned away from the clinical dentistry environment to talk in comparative quiet to assess her difficulties in greater detail. The purpose of the formal psychological assessment was to determine if implant surgery was indicated. On first impression the work seemed to be clearly indicated although the consultants were concerned that the level of distress they encountered may in some way interfere with her ability to recover from the series of surgical operations. It was clear from the physical assessment that she would require bone transplants to build up the maxilla to a level that would enable the osseo-integrated studs to knit properly and to have enough support. The jaw was very thin as a result of bone atrophy from the loss of teeth over a number of years.

During the interview the patient said that she lived with a husband (a retired mechanical engineer) who took very little notice of her and spent most of his time alone in his workshop. She related a history of a poor marriage following a mastectomy some 20 years' earlier, when she had had to sell her beauty therapy business and became fully financially dependent on her husband. She attended outpatient clinics with a scarf around her mouth to prevent others from seeing her face. This woman had many positive qualities: for example, she was very musical and could sing well, accompanied or solo. It was clear from further interviewing that she was depressed. It was difficult, however, to determine whether she was depressed because of her facial appearance – which she rated very low – or as a result of or lack of positive experiences, as she had become something of a recluse. She was recommended for bone transplant and implant retained over dentures with continued follow-up on a regular basis by the clinical psychologist. Over a period of two years' treatment this woman made notable strides in improving her social contacts. She started to attend a local art club and regularly travelled on coach excursions around the region with acquaintances. Her marriage still proved difficult, however she did feel less guilty about leaving her husband to his activities at home. She was very sensitive about her appearance to others and her requests for adjustments to her denture required great patience from the dental surgeons and prosthodontists. The depression experienced by this individual started to lift when she felt able to be seen by others. The treatment of providing implants was beneficial in that the patient was able to feel more comfortable with strangers and acquaintances and therefore socialise more frequently. Her concern for her appearance did not diminish and she showed a sensitised response to any minor changes that occurred during the fitting of the dentures following the surgery phase of her treatment. Close collaboration between the psychologist and consultant prosthodontist ensured that this patient received appropriate treatment.

disfigurement may be summarised under general skills. These are listed as being able to demonstrate:

- Personal warmth
- Self-esteem
- Spontaneity
- Unconditional positive regard
- Empathy
- Genuineness; and
- Not being defensive (Bradbury 1996).

Problems can arise when counselling disfigured individuals due to the clinician who stereotypes and omits to recognise that the person is still an individual. In addition the clinician should be aware of their own reactions to the disfigured individual. Awareness of these reactions will prevent a 'blank' spot in the overall management of the person being treated. This chapter will continue to present some of the factors that social scientists working with dental and medical researchers have identified in understanding people's reactions to facial appearance and possible difficulties.

Facial attractiveness

Case 8c shows that the straightforward dental problem of poor denture fit was only one of many difficulties that the patient experienced. Treatment planning required the health personnel to be sensitive to the patient's depressive feelings (see Chapter 9) and her concern to retain facial attractiveness. In order to make sense of the patient's requests to improve facial appearance it is important to understand society's response to facial appearance. Both psychological and sociological factors are implicated. In 1979, one of the international cosmetic companies had an annual sales figure of $2.38 billion – mainly facial products. The huge investments in the cosmetic industry reflect the level of importance given by members of the public to appearance, especially of the face. Why should people be so concerned with the face? Some reasons are listed:

- Facial information is usually the first that is available.
- It is continuously available during an interaction.

- Physical appearance information does not depend on complex information processing and retrieval.
- Increased incidence of meeting new people, and in situations that may be fleeting.

FACIAL APPEARANCE AND LIKING, DATING AND MARRIAGE

Early research in the 1970s suggested that facial appearance played a major role in liking and dating. More recently, facial appearance has been shown to be important in making friends although other factors such as how similar attitudes were held among friends (i.e. attitude similarity) are also important. The weight of evidence suggests that individuals often marry people of similar physical attractiveness to themselves.

FACIAL APPEARANCE IN PERSUASION, EMPLOYMENT AND ADVERTISING

The social and psychological effects of facial appearance suggest that some aspects of appearance (i.e. attractiveness) may improve ratings and expectations, but there is little evidence that actual behaviour is affected. Other variables may be more important, such as credibility or expertise of the communicator.

FACIAL APPEARANCE AND EDUCATION

On the basis of a child's photograph a sample of 500 teachers were asked to assess the child's IQ, relationship with classmates, parents' attitudes to school and length of time child would remain in full-time education. The attractiveness of the child had a significant positive effect on all four ratings. However, the effects were small and were demonstrable because of the large sample sizes. Children who were highly attractive had a mean IQ of 108 and those of low attractiveness, 106. In practical terms the effect appears to be small.

An important finding has been that teachers underestimate the intelligence of children with cleft palates. However, the extent to which this was a result of the children's speech, rather than the effect of any facial disfigurement, is unknown (Richman 1978).

A study of 320 teachers found their expectations of children did not vary with a child's dental facial appearance. However, whether the teachers had guessed the purpose of the study is arguable, and hence biased their views. The problem of conducting experiments without confounding influences (e.g. participants guessing the reason for the research and altering their responses systematically) is a constant theme in research on facial appearance. Shaw continued his work and examined the effect of perceivers' judgements (for instance, of friendliness, intelligence and aggressiveness), of varying children's dental appearance (by using a photographic superimposition procedure). He found that the variations in dental-facial appearance (i.e. normal, prominent, crowded, missing incisors, or hare lip) had several significant effects. However, he also wisely varied background facial attractiveness and found this to have a stronger effect on ratings. This is an important result for those involved in assisting dental appearance. Patients who have certain attractive facial features, e.g. eyes, will tend to be rated positively on appearance regardless of other less appealing facial features.

Negative reactions to facial disfigurements are acquired by children at about eight years of age. The frequency of teasing in school has been investigated. Among children aged nine to 13, teeth are the fourth most frequent feature to be teased about and give the most distress (Shaw, Meek & Jones 1980). Children do not appear to be aware of the degree of distress they cause and may not purposefully want to cause upset. Unfortunately the chronically teased child can become depressed, socially withdrawn and even suicidal (Gerrard 1991).

Psychological effects of malocclusion

The evidence presented above indicates that facial appearance and to some extent dental appearance do have an effect on relationships and how people judge each other. Those who work in the dental field believe dental appearance to be very important in many real-life situations. It is interesting to see whether this is indeed the case. Rutzen interviewed 252 people five years after an orthodontic treatment had been completed, and compared their data with those of an untreated malocclusion control group. Small and 'barely statistically significant' differences between the two groups were found in occupational rank, in whether married/engaged, in self-assessment of personal appearance, and in anxiety. Factors that did not discriminate included educational level, self-esteem and personality (i.e. neuroticism, extroversion). He concluded that 'the low level of differences may be due to the infrequent use of malocclusion as a basis for social discrimination' (Rutzen 1973).

In 1981, Korabik stated that although many health professionals had noted that improvements in dental appearance led to positive psychological improvements, 'this evidence is anecdotal, and controlled research is needed to confirm their premises'. She asked undergraduates to rate for 'intelligence, morality, adjustment and personal feelings', photographs of adolescent girls' faces (with mouths closed), taken before and after orthodontic treatment. The ratings were summed per photograph to form an 'interpersonal attraction' index, and it was found that the post-orthodontic treatment summated scores differed from the pretreatment scores and from those for the control group (Korabik 1981). Korabik claimed that 'results of this study verify the claim that orthodontic treatment can have psychological as well as physical benefits for those who receive it'. However, this claim is probably going beyond Korabik's evidence. She merely showed that orthodontic treatment affected ratings in an ecologically weak, unrealistic situation (i.e. two-dimensional photographs). Such ratings may not affect behaviour in real-life settings, since interpersonal attraction and other behaviours are the result of a large combination of factors, only one of these being facial appearance. Orthodontic appearance has been found to influence personality ratings, but this effect is less strong than many other aspects of facial appearance especially the eyes (see Shaw's work referred to earlier).

One of the most significant studies to evaluate the psychological and social effects of malocclusion has been conducted by Pamela Kenealy and her co-workers (Kenealy, Frude & Shaw 1989). Ratings of dental status and physical attractiveness, and measures of psychological wellbeing were obtained for a sample of 1018, children aged between 11–12 years old in south Wales. The association between the dentist's rating of malocclusion and the child's ratings of attractiveness and self-esteem was very low showing that there is little support for the major hypothesis that children 'suffer' psychologically from having poor dentition. However, some caution is raised by the authors:

- Although the results fail to support the hypothesis neither do they 'disprove' it.
- The measures may not have been the best to demonstrate the psychological cost of malocclusion.
- Psychological impairment as a result of malocclusion may not become apparent until a later stage in life.
- The result does not impinge on the need for treatment for children with severe malocclusion.

Facial disfigurement

Case 8d   Significance of the face for psychological health

Gender: Male   Age: 20   Occupation: Student

Referral: Secondary referral from orthodontics consultant

Problem: Dissatisfied with reconstructive surgery

Features: Mild cleft palate repaired over stages according to natural development.

This patient was very concerned about his appearance and always attended his sessions at the dental school well groomed and smartly dressed. He was self-conscious about the shape of his upper lip. He wore some camouflage makeup to hide some scarring on the upper lip towards his nostrils. However he was dissatisfied with the outcome and

---

appeared depressed. He was keen to undergo repeated elective surgery from the plastic surgeons to continue to disguise and obliterate all signs of previous surgery. It was explained to the patient that further surgery would not necessarily produce the desired result. The staff within the dental school all regarded him as sociable and well-liked. The patient was very sensitive to his appearance, wondering if people would notice his lip.

The clinical observation that even a small disfigurement can produce significant psychological problems is highlighted by this case. The difficulty for the person with a mild disfigurement lies in the fear that strangers whom they meet will focus on their disfigurement – whereas people with severe disfigurements are not caught in this uncertainty. The uncertainty with the milder disfigurement can lead to a sense of losing some control of the situation and substantially increases anxiety (Lansdown 1990).

The profound social significance of the face, and society's prejudices towards those who have an atypical appearance, can mean that an unattractive facial appearance could be felt as if it was a severe disability. It is difficult to get members of the public to admit prejudice or the social rejection of those with a facial disfigurement. One potent method of determining the behaviour of the public with respect to facially disfigured people is to observe nonverbal communication (for example, eye contact may be avoided or posture may be turned away from disfigured person: see Chapter 6 for a definition of non-verbal behaviour). This approach is likely to be more fruitful than asking for people's opinions by traditional attitude surveys or questionnaires. Many people are not normally conscious of their non-verbal communication. This form of communication is almost automatic and therefore difficult to suppress. Hence, reactions to people with facial disfigurement may be observed better through watching people's non-verbal communication. Ray Bull and his colleagues have demonstrated that the public do avoid people with minor facial disfigurements. Three studies were conducted by Bull's team which

illustrate the potential of disfigurement to shape other's behaviour and are described in Box 8.2 (Bull 1990).

BOX 8.2   EFFECTS OF DISFIGUREMENT ON THE BEHAVIOUR OF OTHERS

Study 1   A female researcher stood on the pavement in a shopping street trying to engage a brief encounter with members of the public. If the researcher had a port-wine stain (using an expert makeup artist to administer a port-wine stain) on her face many members of the public would attempt to avoid her if possible by increasing their pace, averting their gaze and attempting to ignore the presence of the disfigured person. This avoidance is picked up by the disfigured person who frequently interprets it as a form of rejection.

Study 2   A similar design was adopted. Disfigured individuals were compared with individuals of 'normal' appearance, and the research found that more money was placed in a charity box held by the person of 'normal' appearance compared to the disfigured person.

Study 3   A similar design was again used comparing a disfigured with a normal appearance. An individual walked across a pedestrian crossing and it was found that pedestrians stood further away from the disfigured (port-wine stain = 100 cm on average; cuts and bruises = 78 cm) than the non-disfigured person (56 cm).

Orthognathic surgeons have investigated in a series of longitudinal studies the influence of surgical interventions to correct a large range of disfiguring and functional impairments in patients (Kiyak 1993). These studies have clearly shown the benefit of surgical modification to enhance function and appearance. Longitudinal studies to date have shown patients report a marked improvement in self-esteem as well as being satisfied with treatment. These effects appeared to be stable over time and were effective with patients who were of an anxious disposition. These results should reassure clinicians who are cautious about embarking on relatively major surgery with patients showing mild psychological difficulties. The generally anxious patient did have a tendency to complain more about the after-effects of surgery such as pain but the final outcome was regarded from the patient's point of view as positive. In summary, the orthognathic evidence shows the clear benefit of corrective modification but this is more difficult to demonstrate in milder conditions such as maloccluded dentition. It should be noted however that these results are based upon group comparison. The individual variation of responses to malocclusion may be high and therefore an individual approach to each patient is important when conducting assessment. However, facial disfigurement (even minor instances) would appear to have fairly major effects on people's behaviour judged by some naturalistic studies. This is also demonstrated by this chapter's fourth case (Case 8d) where a high level of self-reported dissatisfaction was found with a mild disfigurement of the upper lip. The research in this field does require a significant boost to avoid basing clinical judgements and health service provision solely on anecdotal reports. It is hoped that longitudinal studies will provide us with the much needed information to improve knowledge and treatment.

References

Backett K 1990 Studying health in families: a qualitative approach. In: Cunningham-Burley S, McKeganey N (eds.) Readings in Medical Sociology London: Tavistock/Routledge

Blinkhorn A 1989 Promoting dietary changes in order to control dietary caries. Journal of the Institute of Health Education 27:179–186

Blinkhorn A 1993 Compliance with dental regimens. International Dental Journal 43(3):294–298

Bradbury E 1996 Counselling people with disfigurement. Leicester: British Psychological Society

Bull R H C 1990 Society's reaction to facial disfigurements. Dental Update (June) 202–205

Gerrard J 1991 The teasing syndrome in facially deformed children. Australian and New Zealand Journal of Family Therapy 12:147–154

Graham H 1985 Caring for the family. Milton Keynes: Open University

Graham H 1993 Hardship and health in women's lives. London: Harvester Wheatsheaf

Grytten J, Rostow I, Steele L, Holst D 1988 Aspects of the formation of dental health behaviours in early childhood. Journal of the Institute of Health Education, 26(2):62–68

Holmes T H, Rahe R H 1967 The social readjustment ratings scale. Journal of Psychosomatic Research 11:213–218

Kay E, McGuiness J 1990 Pregnant women's dental health knowledge. Dental Health 29(2):3–5

Kenealy P, Frude N, Shaw W 1989 An evaluation of the psychological and social effects of malocclusion: some implications for dental policy making. Social Science and Medicine 28:59–65

Kiyak H 1993 Psychological aspects of orthognathic surgery. Special issue: dental health psychology. Psychology and Health, 8(2–3):197–212

Korabik K 1981 Changes in physical attractiveness and interpersonal attraction. Basic and Applied Social Psychology 2:59–65

Lansdown R 1990 Psychological problems of patients with cleft lip and palate: discussion paper. Journal of the Royal Society of Medicine 83:448–450

Richman L 1978 The effects of facial disfigurement on teachers' perception of ability in cleft palate children. Cleft Palate Journal 15:155–160

Rutzen S 1973 The social importance of orthodontic rehabilitation: report on a five year follow-up study. Journal of Health and Social Behaviour 14:233–240

Shaw W C, Meek S C, Jones D S 1980 Nicknames, teasing, harassment and the salience of dental features among school children. British Journal of Orthodontics 7:75–80

Symmonds A 1991 Angels and interfering busybodies: the social construction of two occupations. Sociology of Health and Illness 13(2):249–264

9

Psychosocial reactions and oral health disorders

Case 9a Interrelated general and dental health problems

Gender: Female   Age: 19   Occupation: Unemployed

Referral: From local general dental practitioner

Problem: Dental phobia with concerns over dental appearance (dysmorphophobia)

Features:Assistance was required from GDP to help patient accept dental treatment. Patient was already receiving treatment for depression from local health services.

On initial interview this woman appeared very agitated and expressed not only difficulties about receiving dental treatment but also an acute self-consciousness over her two top incisors which she regarded as very prominent. She also related that she was an outpatient at the local psychiatric day centre receiving supportive psychotherapy from one of the ward staff (a psychiatric nurse). Contact was made with the outpatient unit to determine the nature of the treatment she received and the nature of her difficulties. She had suffered a bout of depression recently and was making good progress, taking a mild anxiolytic prior to going to bed at night. It was agreed with the outpatient unit that she should attend the clinical psychologist's office initially and start some desensitisation to dental objects including the syringe and the drill handpiece. After a couple of sessions the dental school was informed that she had taken an overdose and had been admitted to a psychiatric ward. Three months later she

made a dental visit after suffering an acute abscess which required emergency treatment under general anaesthesia. Following her GA visit she returned to see the clinical psychologist. Discussion focused on whether there was a link between her embarking on a programme of dental treatment and her sudden depressive relapse and overdose. She felt that the opportunity to start becoming more familiar with dental instruments and then get used to the dental surgery just prior to attempting an examination in the dental chair was both hopeful, but also daunting. She very much wanted to receive treatment for her front teeth and was willing herself to succeed in starting dental treatment properly. However the prospect of failure was also a feature of this approach to receiving treatment. The fear of failure was an important element in promoting her lowly self-image ('what will happen if I don't manage to receive dental treatment after all this effort, then I will be really useless'). These negative statements strengthened her depressive feelings about herself and the influence of a recently failed relationship prompted her to take an overdose. Recognition of the potential for negative self-statements to influence mood and generate thoughts of self-destruction were an important part of this patient re-entering the process of systematic desensitisation and eventual successful dental treatment. Her front teeth were filled but tooth size remained unaltered. The concern about her appearance was not a persistent

> symptom following her sessions which
> included discussion of her depression and the
> reasons for her mood changes.

This case demonstrates a number of valuable points:

1. Dental phobia may be only one of a number of psychological difficulties that a patient presents with.
2. The professional boundaries between staff from different disciplines must not interfere with accurate and timely exchange of information about a patient's condition. It was fortunate in this case that good contacts had been made prior to the overdose so that an efficient exchange of opinions could flow between the parties concerned.
3. The importance of constructing a formulation which includes the major features of the patient's condition and exploration of the relations between them by adopting a model (in this case a cognitive formulation) to point towards suitable management.

This case therefore draws on many of the conditions that are presented in this chapter including dental phobia, body dysmorphophobic disorder, depression, anorexia and body image. Although she would not match all the criteria for each of these mental health problems, knowledge of them would nevertheless assist the clinician in choice of treatment approach and general management.

In clinical practice in whatever service sector (public, private or hospital) a wide variety of patients will be seen with a range of both physical and psychological problems. A substantial minority will be experiencing more extreme psychological difficulties which may be termed 'psychological disorders'. Other terms exist such as 'psychological dysfunction'. These descriptions of mental health problems will tend to overlap with psychiatric terms which emphasise conditions with mental illness as its focus. This book does not use a traditional psychiatric system of classifying mental health problems. The majority of dental patients can be helped by using a psychological explanation to indicate management. Such an approach is often

preferred by patients. A psychiatric system of assessment and treatment related to dental practice has been compiled (Enoch & Jagger 1994) in which rarer and unusual cases are presented. The purpose of this chapter is to focus on:

- The more common problems that may be encountered in dental practice;
- Links between physical and mental health problems; and
- implications for clinical management.

Psychological distress related to pain and fear of the dentist

In a recent survey of over 800 UK dental attenders it was found that 27% of patients showed at least one symptom of psychological distress (Green et al. 1997). The sample was collected from nine dental practices throughout England, Wales and Scotland. Psychological distress was assessed by the General Health Questionnaire which has been employed extensively in primary care settings. The 12-question version was used which made it suitable for use in a busy surgery (there are 28; 30- and 60-question versions of this measure). The 27% of respondents who reported three or more symptoms are considered to need, or alternatively would benefit from, some form of psychological or psychiatric help. It was found that many of these patients were afraid or in dental pain. It is unclear as yet whether the experience of dental pain or being anxious about the dentist precipitates general distress or alternatively the distress itself increases dental pain and anxiety. Of particular interest in this study was the extensive range (18–51%) in distress levels across practices.

A possible explanation for the differences between practices may be that patients self-select their dentist on the basis of personal recommendation. They seek out those dental practices which may have a more or less sensitive approach to other concerns of patients such as how they feel generally. Some patients may prefer a straightforward, clearly focused and treatment-orientated service which tends not to focus on additional issues; other patients are comfortable with an indirect approach which enables other patient difficulties to be tolerated and possibly expressed during the course of dental care provided by their chosen dentist. It is worth speculating why there should be such a large variation in distress across practices. Does the dentist allow patients to express their worries so that patients relax and accept treatment? Do patients find the visit much more pleasant than they had expected and are they therefore more likely to attend that dentist? It may be that the dentist's working relationship encourages a certain type of patient to attend.

This theme of trying to determine causality is a thread that runs through many of the dental conditions with a psychological aspect to their etiology and maintenance.

The rest of this chapter presents a number of conditions seen in patients with dental problems which have psychological features that may contribute indirectly to the difficulties that the person experiences. In some cases the influence of psychological factors may impinge directly on the dental complaint.

The first three conditions – Temperomandibular Joint (TMJ) Pain Dysfunction Syndrome, Bruxism and Burning Mouth Syndrome – are examples where similar causes are implicated: 'stress' in a patient's life for instance is regarded as a possible factor to explain the condition. The patient's personality is another important area to investigate, although each of the three conditions has its own specific etiology. This provides a fascinating example of how conditions focused around the mouth have generated a variety of methods and approaches. The extent that socio-psychological explanations are involved is unfortunately difficult to quantify, but it is a useful clinical skill to have an awareness of possible factors that could help understand a patient's presenting problems. Careful questioning and gathering of information by listening to patients will do a great deal to assess the importance of additional elements that feature in patients' description of their symptoms.

Temperomandibular joint pain dysfunction syndrome (PDS)

This condition has been defined as the presence of one or more of the following signs and symptoms: pain and tenderness in the region of the masticatory muscles of the temperomandibular joint (TMJ), clicking or crepitation of the TMJ during condylar movement and limitation of mandibular movement. PDS is also termed facial arthromyalgia, myogenic facial pain, myofascial pain dysfunction syndrome as well as other related forms of words.

Case 9b Is personality involved in causing or maintaining jaw pain?

Gender: Female   Age: 45   Occupation: Part-time teacher

Referral: From local general dental practitioner

Problem: Chronic TMJ pain

Features: Generally anxious as well as fearful of doing permanent damage to jaw.

A woman of 45 was referred to the dental teaching hospital with TMJ pain. There was little visible organic involvement and the patient was seen for cognitive behavioural treatment. She was married with a young son; her difficulty stemmed from the time when she had married some five years earlier and started a family. She was particularly keen to understand whether the pain she experienced was psychological in origin. Her greatest fear was clenching or clamping her jaw on some solid food which would permanently damage her jaw. She hoped that her pain would be understood from factors such as the pressure she felt from a demanding job teaching gifted children and looking after a demanding and 'clingy' child. She described herself as neurotic and prone to stress – her self-esteem was low and she felt depressed and hopeless about the future.

This patient matches the features that are believed to be involved in this condition. PDS is of multifactorial origin and is a result of a combination of occlusal, neurophysiological and psychological factors. A study by Laan et al. (1988) confirmed that in a group of TMJ patients ($n = 261$), some with complete dentition and others with a complete upper and lower denture, a whole set of psychological variables were correlated to the dysfunction of the TMJ. These variables included neuroticism, pessimism or negativism and somatisation (that is, the tendency to complain with bodily symptoms where no organic evidence can be found).

Many studies of this type have been reported. A problem in explaining the patient's experience is that many personality factors have been implicated, and as a clinician it is difficult to know which one to focus on. Chronic pain may change the personality of a patient, and therefore the direction of cause and effect may be reversed. Having said this, many clinicians are convinced that the personality of a patient may cause a susceptibility to experiencing pain, and this possible mechanism should be considered in treating patients. For example, a generally anxious patient may benefit from inspecting which areas of her life are causing the distress, and be able to make changes which help to relieve her long-term concerns. Referral to registered or chartered therapists (counsellors, psychotherapists or clinical psychologists) may be warranted.

Sociologists have identified that health professionals as a social group tend to focus on explanations that suit the profession as opposed to the patient that the group is employed to help. To prevent preconceived ideas unduly influencing the attempts to understand this group of patients there is a role for listening at length to patients' conversations about their problems. An interesting study by Linda Garro uses in-depth interviews (see Chapter 11 for more detail about this research method) to investigate 32 TMJ sufferers. She concentrates on encouraging her study participants to recount their experiences of TMJ (Garro 1994). It is clear from the analysis of these 'stories' that chronic symptoms are not amenable to simple categorisation. Attempts to fit patient experiences into the models of care currently offered by health services were only partially successful. Of great concern for those

interviewed was whether their pain or dysfunction was a result of physical or psychological factors. When the pattern of symptoms does not match expectations held by others (spouses, friends, doctors or dentists) then their concerns are highlighted. The implications of this study for clinicians is to encourage them to listen to the patient's description of her problem carefully, then attempt to match the patient's explanation, as closely as possible, to the clinician's own assessment from physical examination and any additional test results available.

When a joint acceptance of a formulation for the patient's problem has been agreed a treatment plan can be prepared. Some evidence for selecting different therapies to suit patients with different profiles has been reported. In a pool of 57 patients with chronic TMJ pain, relaxation was compared with biofeedback therapy. Those who benefited from relaxation therapy tended to be younger, had suffered pain for a shorter duration and reported other psychophysiologic disorders (Funch & Gale 1984). Biofeedback especially benefited older married patients who had the TMJ pain for longer and who had already received treatment to correct their occlusion.

Clinicians have reported depression to be a marked feature of PDS although empirical studies are mixed in support of this common clinical report. Depression may be recognised by apathy, a poor estimate of self-worth, poor compliance and indecisiveness as well as low mood and tearfulness. Depression is treatable and a recommendation to the patient to visit their general medical practitioner is advocated. A recent study has argued for making a distinction in patients with PDS between those with and without a mental disorder (Morris et al. 1997). Of the 97 patients investigated 32 (33%) had a mental disorder. Splitting PDS patients into this dichotomy assists its management. These authors were able to present findings which supported the view that 'psychosocial factors contribute to the presentation and possible causation of PDS' in the group of patients with identifiable mental disorder. This view may be controversial, however psychological factors and the possibility of mental difficulties should be considered especially if conventional physical approaches to treatment do not assist progress.

BOX 9.1 CLINICAL IMPLICATIONS WHEN TREATING TMJ PATIENTS

- Assess physical aetiology thoroughly.
- If there is significant evidence for a physical explanation of symptoms, listen to the patient's account/description of the problem.
- Note that although the personality of the patient may exacerbate the symptoms it may also be the case that personality characteristics are concentrated to a greater extent by clinicians looking for an expedient theory.
- Assess for depression (simple scales such as the Hospital Anxiety and Depression Scale may be used). If a high level of depressive symptoms is found suggest that the patient discusses how he feels with his medical practitioner.

Bruxism

There are numerous clinical reports and theoretical papers which suggest that nocturnal oral muscle hyperactivity or the 'non-functional clenching and grinding of teeth' known as bruxism is related to a number of different variables including psychological factors. Measurement of bruxism has been varied and includes: self-report questionnaires, diary keeping by the partner, electromyography in which electrodes are placed over the masseter muscle blocks while the person sleeps, intraoral transmitters and tooth wear. The operational definitions of bruxism have often not been provided in these clinical reports. Nocturnal and diurnal bruxism should be distinguished as it is likely that different factors are implicated in the two forms.

What are the causes of bruxism? Four principal theories are believed to account for the condition:

1. Some evidence has been reported to link nocturnal bruxism with different stages of the sleep cycle. Patients who had severe symptoms known as 'destructive' bruxers were found to exhibit more bruxism during Rapid Eye Movement sleep than a group of bruxers who also complained from sleep disturbance (Ware & Rugh 1988).
2. Drug use, both illicit and prescribed, has been suggested as a factor to explain bruxism. A drug side-effect has been noted by authors from north Wales and reported by others: they have identified the development of bruxism in patients prescribed one of the newer antidepressants known as serotonin reuptake inhibitors (SSRIs). In one patient they report a dose–response curve with the amount of tooth grinding (Fitzgerald & Healy 1995). A recent phenomenon to add to the list of causative factors of which the clinician should be aware when examining a patient who shows evidence of bruxing (taking tooth wear as a simple indicator) is the influence of taking the drug Ecstasy (methylenedioxymethamphetamine or MDMA) which has become popular among younger people attending nightclubs and rave parties. Associated complaints include frequent headaches, lower back problems and nausea (Cohen 1995).
3. Personality has been favoured as an explanation for bruxism occurring in some patients and not others. Bruxers were found to be 'shy, stiff, cautious, and aloof, preferring things rather than people, avoiding compromises, rigid ... and given to worrying' (Fischer & O'Toole 1993).
4. Stress appears to exacerbate bruxism although there is often an occlusal disparity which contributes to the initial onset (Morse 1982). Patients fitted with a device (electromyogram) to measure muscle activity were found to clench their teeth more during emotionally arousing situations such as driving, having an important meeting, etc.

A large number of treatments have been tested and can be divided into physical and psychological. The physical methods included the manufacture of a mouthguard or splint to wear at night while asleep. The physical barrier will assist in protecting the teeth during sleep. Some patients are unable to tolerate wearing the splint at night, or find it unhelpful. Psychological methods include:

- Biofeedback. Electrodes are taped to lie over the

masseter muscles on either side of the face, and are connected to equipment which translates any high electrical activity from the muscle group, indicating clenching of the jaw, to an amplifier and loudspeaker to produce an alarm.

- Hypnosis.
- Behavioural approaches such as:
  — Relaxation training. A standard relaxation programme could be offered where the clinician talks through the procedure of relaxation exercises with the patient and provides an audiotape cassette of instructions and advice for the patient to use at home – research indicates that relaxation exercises taught from an audiocassette alone are not very effective.
  — Aversive conditioning. An example of this approach would be an extension of biofeedback to include a very high pitched alarm sound. The approach may be indicated for use with nocturnal bruxers where repeated waking from sleep would prove aversive. Such an approach would only be used with the explicit permission of the patient, full explanation of the purpose of such methods and where other less extreme approaches had not proved successful.

A comparison study of suggested treatments – stress-reducing behavioural counselling and nocturnal biofeedback – with a waiting list control showed that the stress reduction procedure was more effective than biofeedback, although all interventions were better than the no-treatment waiting list control condition (Casas, Beemsterboer & Clark 1982).

BOX 9.2   CLINICAL IMPLICATIONS OF TREATING THE PATIENT WHO SUFFERS BRUXISM

- Assess for stressful life events or general level of 'hassle'
- Assess medication and recreational drug use
- Determine what approaches patients have already tried

- Refer to general medical practitioner, counselling, psychotherapy or clinical psychology service.

Burning mouth syndrome

Case 9c   'Pain has many uses'

Gender: Female   Age: 34   Occupation: Part-time personal assistant

Referral: From local general dental practitioner
Problem: Burning Mouth Syndrome
Features: A burning pain felt on the left side of the tongue and cheek which was triggered by contact with tooth that had been restored.

A female patient of 34 was referred from the oral medicine unit of a dental teaching hospital following the standard battery of physical examinations and physiological tests (i.e. blood tests, saliva analysis) which proved normal. She was seen by the clinical psychologist for 20 sessions. The patient was married to an Asian financial broker and had two children aged two and four years. She was currently working as a housewife and as a part-time assistant to the head of a law firm. When she worked full-time she had been the personal assistant to the managing director of a manufacturing business, where she had met her husband. She felt a great deal of pain from the left side of her mouth which was triggered when she 'caught' her tongue against a lower mandibular molar tooth which had recently been restored with a crown. She had made repeated visits to her local general dental practitioner who polished the surface of the crown and surrounding teeth. The patient was compelled to inspect her mouth daily to determine if the tooth and the tongue showed evidence of irregularities and would ask her husband to check for her as well as her dentist. She stated that the pain

---

from the left side of her mouth prevented her from enjoying life and she feared that the catching of her tongue would not disappear until the offending tooth had been entirely remodelled. This difficulty had prevented her from continuing with some of her usual household and social activities, and the experience of pain was generally dampening her enjoyment of life.

After discussion with the patient and an examination of her pain diary it became clear that her pain complaints enabled a closer relationship to be maintained between the couple as she would ask for assistance in checking her mouth and ask for reassurance. She was also very bored with staying at home and keen to return to work full-time. Her husband held more traditional values and was adamant that she should continue looking after their children full-time, but he was caring of her facial discomfort and did try to understand. A response prevention approach was taken. The patient was advised not to check her tooth for irregularities or ask her husband to assist her in this.
Recommendations were made to the couple to engage in more activities (family and social), to share responsibilities and positive experiences. Hence a formulation was

generated from the interviews which supported the view that the wife's condition was associated to family and occupational factors requiring acknowledgement and change in both husband and wife. The diagram of the pain diary scores is reproduced in Fig. 9.1 and shows the gradual change and lowering of self-reported pain level over an extended period of some months.

The case above is an example of a condition referred to as Burning Mouth Syndrome (BMS). It presents in a variety of guises and the case presented is not entirely typical. Burning Mouth Syndrome is a set of burning and painful sensations in the mouth when investigation of the clinical mucosa proves normal. The incidence of BMS is approximately 3% of the population (Mott, Grushka & Sessle 1993) and characteristically patients are surprised that others suffer from their complaint, as they have no general knowledge of the condition. A large number of causative agents have been proposed including:

- Local (for example, dental materials used for making dentures)
- Systemic including the lack of minerals, vitamins etc.

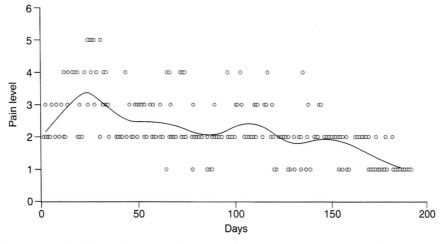

Fig. 9.1 Patient's self-reported daily pain diary as rated on a 1 to 10 scale, where 1 is 'no pain' and 10 is 'pain as bad as it can be' collected over 190 days. A 'smoothed' curve has been fitted to the data points for ease of interpretation.

- Stressful life events
- Mental health problems
- Social difficulties.

Psychopharmacological treatment is often offered to BMS sufferers including antidepressants. Patients who opt for this form of medication do not however always get relief – either they find the side effects (e.g. drowsiness) difficult to cope with, or they report some relief but are then troubled with a dry mouth which is also difficult to manage. Drug side-effects can diminish with time although some patients are not prepared to continue with medication.

BOX 9.3   COGNITIVE BEHAVIOUR THERAPY

A cognitive behavioural approach is used to assist explanation of those conditions where appropriate physical diagnosis is not available. There is a risk of attributing a psychological reason to a patient whose symptom is not diagnosable because of:

- The unavailability of a suitable test
- An error in physical examination
- An assessment conducted during a 'recovery' period which did not confirm an organic explanation.

It is important to appreciate that the public are prepared to accept physical explanations of disease but are reluctant to believe that psychological factors may assist diagnosis. Therefore the clinician should be careful in explaining to patients that their dento-facial problem may have some other causes apart from the physical. As a theoretical position the cognitive behavioural therapy approach is currently the most popular as the perspective that is able to contribute to our understanding and offer empirical demonstrable interventions. The ability to incorporate an individual's thoughts, feelings and behaviour, the consequences of that behaviour and physiological processes in a social context is a powerful approach, used judiciously, to assist understanding of the sufferer, and provide therapeutic techniques that facilitate changes

---

in thinking (to correct irrational or unrealistic thoughts) and behaviour (i.e. reduce avoidance such as isolating oneself from social activities) as well as offering alternative methods of coping with anxiety-provoking situations. The dental member of staff adopting the skills presented in Chapter 6 (especially listening skills) should be able to assess the dental patient and reach a decision to seek further referral, either to the patient's general medical practitioner or to a specialist centre such as the dental teaching hospital.

An alternative psychological approach may be adopted (Humphris, Longman & Field 1996) which is called Cognitive Behaviour Therapy (CBT). The term 'cognitive behavioural' is explained in Box 9.3. The CBT approach consists of four elements:

1. Assessment
2. Formulation
3. Intervention
4. Behavioural change.

Assessment is required to get a detailed history of the patient's pain experience to determine its duration, frequency and course. A useful tool is the completion of a daily pain diary (mentioned in Chapter 7) where the patient completes a simple 1–10 rating scale of the peak level of pain experienced coupled with any brief comments alongside the rating of a significant event that occurred that day or a particular concern of which the patient was aware. An example from a patient record is presented in Fig. 9.1 that clearly demonstrates a temporal link between events and pain level. It is also imperative to access what beliefs the patient has about the episodes and causes of their pain and whether they feel they have the ability to change their pain or adopt a particular method to cope with it. Deriving a formulation to help explain or at least co-ordinate all this information into a coherent order assists both clinician and patient to test out various hypotheses of what may change the patient's pain experience. Finally, an intervention to change some of the habitual and perhaps unhelpful behavioural and thinking patterns that the patient has adopted over months and perhaps years is implemented with the co-operation of the patient who is involved at every level. The major aim then of this form of psychotherapy is to modify some of the 'automatic negative thinking patterns' which alter behavioural responses to pain (e.g. avoiding social occasions).

CBT (sometimes referred to just as Cognitive Therapy) has been found to be effective (Bergdahl, Anneroth & Perris 1995) with resistant BMS patients (that is, those who had some medication but without success). On a measure of BMS intensity – an 8 point rating scale that ranged from endurable to unendurable – found that the group (n = 15) receiving cognitive therapy showed a significant improvement (reduction in rating from 5 to 2) in their condition – this was found post treatment to have been maintained for six months. The attentional/placebo group showed no change in intensity of burning sensations. These authors cited their results as demonstrating that in some cases resistant BMS was psychogenic in origin. Clinical trials to compare drug and cognitive behaviour therapies (including both approaches combined as one of the arms of the trial) are being completed and their results eagerly awaited. This area of oral health is gaining interest as both the profession and the public gain in knowledge about the problems associated with BMS.

The osseo-integrated implant field

Patients who lose their teeth and become edentulous tend to have difficulty in retaining their dentures as the supportive bony ridge of both jaws is absorbed gradually over time. The introduction of titanium pins screwed directly into the remaining jawbone to act as supportive structures to assist the retention of an overdenture is now a routine procedure although careful surgical assessment and regular follow-up is required. Psychological assessment is also recommended in some cases: studies in Sheffield and Liverpool have shown that a small group of patients suffered considerable psychological distress following this treatment (Humphris et al. 1995; Kent & Johns 1993). It is unclear whether surgical intervention may have a

bearing on these few patients' mental state. Kent and Johns suggest that this patient group tend to be elderly and therefore may be facing a number of significant life events such as bereavement, retirement or relocation – the psychological distress being monitored is therefore independent of the dental treatment. Humphris et al. have put forward a psychobiological explanation. Patients with substantial bone loss (and so a more severe physical problem) have expectations that may not be as great as those with moderate bone loss. It was found that those experiencing psychological distress and poor self-esteem together with dissatisfaction about their mouths were from the category of only moderate bone loss. This is interesting as this moderate bone loss group would have been marginal for selection of treatment as their physical need was less.

BOX 9.4   CLINICAL IMPLICATIONS WHEN TREATING IMPLANT PATIENTS AND THOSE WHO RECEIVE IRREVERSIBLE SPECIALIST AND INVASIVE TREATMENTS

- Patients should be questioned about any significant events they have recently experienced.
- What effect have these experiences had on the patient?
- Estimate how the patient feels generally including their mood and wellbeing.
- Obtain an assessment of patient expectations of the treatment procedure.

Eating disorders

Both men and women experience eating disorders with dental consequences that the observant dentist can assess. Through sensitive interviewing, the patient may be encouraged to recognise that they may need professional help (Milosevic & Slade 1989).

ANOREXIA NERVOSA

The incidence of anorexia nervosa is increasing. A survey in Scotland from 1978–82 estimates the incidence as approximately four persons per 100 000, which is over double the rate calculated for the late 1960s. It has been reported that the female to male ratio is 20:1. Features include refusal to maintain body weight, fear of gaining weight, claims of feeling fat and an absence (in women only) of three consecutive menstrual cycles (amenorrhea). The psychological framework for understanding anorexia can be simplified as follows. An excessive sense of dissatisfaction with herself and perfectionism drives the individual to focus on success in controlling her own body weight. Success is reinforcing and includes a downward spiral of weight loss leading to the serious condition of anorexia.

BULIMIA NERVOSA

More recently a further form of eating disorder has been identified which is characterised by cycles of binge eating followed by self-induced vomiting or the excessive use of laxatives. Some authorities claim that bulimia is more common than anorexia. A study of USA college students recorded a 35% level of incidence. A more representative sample (women at a UK Family Planning Clinic) showed a 2% level of incidence. Features of bulimia include repeated binge-eating episodes, a lack of control over eating behaviour during a binge, stimulus-induced vomiting (SIV), use of laxatives, diuretics and excessive exercise, and at least two binges per week in a three-month period.

From recent evidence dental features include an acid saliva and some increase in gingivitis and plaque levels. The bulimic with a long history of SIV (that is, a total life-history of 1100 or more vomiting episodes) will show marked evidence of characteristic tooth wear due to digestive stomach acids.

Phobic response to dentistry

Extreme dental anxiety, referred to as dental phobia, has been mentioned in Chapter 6 and has generated a great deal of interest in attempts to explain its etiology. The effect of the individual's personality upon the degree of dental fear has been a focus of debate. Some reports associate general anxiety to dental anxiety with mixed results. One report studying extreme dentally anxious patients has found that they show features of insecurity (Schuurs 1988). The best approach for these patients was broad-based, offering a variety of methods to suit their particular difficulty. To strengthen this clinical management approach a categorical distinction between four types of dental phobia has been adopted in a large dental-fear clinic in Seattle, USA (Moore, Brodsgard & Birn 1991):

- A conditioned fear to a specific painful or unpleasant stimulus e.g. needles, drills, sounds or smells.
- Anxiety about a somatic response such as an allergic reaction to the local anaesthetic, fainting or a panic attack. Some of these features relate closely to an agoraphobic condition in which the person has a strong anxiety reaction to strange and unpredictable environments.
- Associated generalised anxiety disorders (GADs) or multiple phobias.
- Distrust of dental personnel associated with social phobias.

The second type of dental phobia referred to above highlights a management problem which requires additional understanding to the simple fear conditioning model (that is, fears precipitated by traumatic event). Patients who are keenly aware of their bodily sensations and who attempt to attend a dentist may suffer a panic attack that is extremely aversive in its own right, in addition to their fear of the dentist or dental surgery. Hence the expression 'fear of fear itself'. These individuals will avoid attendance for the primary reason of preventing a panic attack, so that the dental stimuli (e.g. needles, syringes etc.) become secondary in importance. One perspective that has assisted our understanding of the processes involved in the generation of a panic attack and how patients may be helped has been outlined by the cognitive psychologist Clark and applied to the dental situation, by Barsby (1997). Hyperventilation (over-breathing in the form of very rapid, irregular breaths or sometimes very deep sighs) is an automatic response to certain threatening stimuli that occur in the dental situation (Barsby 1997). The over-breathing rapidly produces a range of symptoms that includes palpitations, tingling, dizziness, derealisation, sweating, trembling, faintness and nausea. The discomfort of these symptoms encourages the individual to focus on possible explanations for them, however the rapidity and the meaning associated with some of these sensations introduces thinking patterns which overestimate the degree of threat (from the sensation) to the individual. In other words, the person interprets his reactions catastrophically ('if this thumping in my chest gets any worse then I really will be in danger of a heart attack'). This thought process, of believing the sensations to be life-threatening, will if unchecked increase anxiety and therefore the desire to inflate the lungs frequently, producing a further decrease in arterial tension of CO_2, which in turn develops stronger body sensations. If allowed to continue this cycle of events will precipitate a panic attack. Two steps are advocated in the dental situation:

STEP 1: RE-ESTABLISH NORMAL ALVEOLAR CARBON DIOXIDE LEVELS

This is achieved by inviting the patient to cup their hands over their nose and mouth and re-breathe their own exhaled air. According to Barsby the simple instruction to breathe regularly and smoothly is often all that is required. With the crisis over the dentist should discuss with the patient the events as they unfolded and explain them. It is helpful to listen to the patient's specific, experienced sensations so that an individualised response is presented to the patient. A hyperventilation test may be conducted in which the patient (after permission has been gained) is instructed to breathe deeply and rapidly (30 breaths per minute) over a two-minute duration. A demonstration can be given by the dentist beforehand. The symptoms produced in the patient can be discussed and parallels drawn between the symptoms felt and those recalled in the dental situation. The patient is encouraged to understand the similarity between sensations produced by the test and receiving dental treatment.

STEP 2: TRAIN THE PATIENT TO LEARN A MORE RELAXED ABDOMINAL FORM OF BREATHING PATTERN

Barsby suggests that patients should place one hand on their chests and the other on their stomach. Breathing should continue at a slow and regular pace (8–10 breaths per minute) with only the stomach moving, therefore restricting chest movement. This method is straightforward and is especially applicable for anxious dental patients who suffer from 'gagging'.

Depression

This condition is common and all dentists are likely to see patients who are depressed (Beck, Kaul & Weaver 1979). It is not known whether patients with depression will tend not to register with a dentist or just feel unable to attend even when they have made an appointment. According to Beck and his colleagues, a survey in the USA reported a one-year prevalence rate of 15% of the adult population. Depression may be recognised from psychological and physical perspectives. Feeling low, an inability to experience pleasure, a sense of worthlessness and difficulty in making decisions are common symptoms of the depressed individual. Physical manifestations include lack of appetite for food and sexual relations, tiredness and a fitful sleeping pattern. Should patients state that they do not feel their life is worth living, – that is, giving an indication of suicidal intention – then this must be taken seriously and the patient encouraged to visit their general medical practitioner without delay. Suicide rates vary across national boundaries: in the UK the suicide rate (in 1990) was 8.1 per 100 000. Attempted suicides have been estimated to be about ten times the suicide rate. Hopelessness is a common feature of an individual who may consider suicide (Lester 1997). The best predictor of suicide is the person who makes their suicide intention known to another. The dental signs when treating a severely depressed patient include the patient's preference for not making a series of protracted visits for intricate treatment or a rapid deterioration in their oral hygiene. Alternatively the patient may request intricate treatment in order to have greater individual attention, although this is likely to be among less severely depressed patients. Unfortunately the assessment of depression from observation of patient responses within the dental surgery is poorly researched.

Obsessions and delusions

Occasionally a patient may be seen who has a strong desire for a perfect dentition, a perfectly fitting denture or perfect oral hygiene, and who is dissatisfied with all the clinician's attempts (maybe after many visits) at assistance. There may be a simple explanation which the patient will volunteer, but sometimes their behaviour can appear obsessive especially if the patient shows signs of irrationality that interfere with everyday behaviour.

Extreme psychological reaction to a feature of body appearance has been termed dysmorphophobia. Morselli in 1886 (as cited by Cunningham et al. 1996) defined this term as 'the sudden onset and subsequent persistence of an idea of deformity; the individual fears he (sic) has become or may become deformed and feels tremendous anxiety of such an awareness'. The DSM-IV (Diagnosis and Statistical Manual, fourth edition, a recognised classification system for psychiatric conditions) has split dysmorphophobia into delusional and non-delusional variants (American Psychological Association 1995). The non-delusional dysmorphophobics are now referred to as persons with Body Dysmorphic Disorder (BDD). Characteristics of BDD include a preoccupation with a defect in appearance which is either imagined or concern over which is excessive. The preoccupation causes substantial distress in social and occupational relationships and cannot be explained by reference to other mental health problems (for example, anorexia nervosa). The delusional form is classified as a psychotic disorder (Cunningham et al. 1996).

It is not easy to give an estimate of the incidence of BDD. This is because many patients with BDD see their problem as purely physical requiring some essential surgical intervention. This view is confirmed by the average duration from 'symptoms' to referral, which is about six years. However the difficulties experienced in maintaining a normal social life are great and considerable time and effort is expended by the person in hiding their presumed defect from others via makeup, camouflage or purely avoiding social situations altogether. Persons with BDD may, in order to obtain surgery, trawl a wide catchment area for a second opinion to locate a sympathetic clinician to perform their operation. Hence careful and observant assessment is required to assist the patient and avoid unnecessary surgery. Surgical intervention is not indicated with minor defects in these individuals and can indeed exacerbate their problem. Formal assessment should be considered and will involve either a clinical psychologist or psychiatrist. A discussion with the patient's general medical practitioner would be important before referral to a specialist. A commonly associated condition is depression which may be a result of avoiding social contact and is of course treatable. It is unlikely that the person who initially suffers depression will become more prone to BDD, although this causative pathway cannot entirely be discounted. Depression may make individuals more vulnerable to criticism and make it more difficult for them to dismiss negative evaluations of themselves. However why a deliberate focus should arise on one aspect of body image remains unknown. Treatment of BDD can be difficult and lengthy. Various options are available, and include cognitive behavioural psychotherapy (Rosen, Reiter & Orosan 1995), pharmacological treatments (Cunningham et al. 1996) and psychoanalytical psychotherapy (Kells et al. 1996).

Practical implications for the dental surgery

- Be observant of patient behaviour.
- Don't be too quick to sum up a patient.
- Give the patient an opportunity to explain unusual behaviour.
- If you suspect there is a problem which is interfering with routine dental care then check patient history, e.g. medication, past hospitalisation.

- Invite the patient to comment on his behaviour/situation. Ask if he wishes to seek advice and suggest he sees his general medical practitioner.
- In the rare event that patients indicate suicidal intent, always treat this seriously.

References

American Psychological Association 1995 Diagnostic and statistical manual of mental disorders, DSM-IV. Washington, DC: American Psychiatric Association

Barsby M 1997 The control of hyperventilation in the management of 'gagging'. British Dental Journal 182(3):109–111

Beck F M, Kaul T J, Weaver J M 1979 Recognition and management of the depressed dental patient. Journal of the American Dental Association 99:967–971

Bergdahl J, Anneroth G, Perris H 1995 Cognitive therapy in the treatment of patients with resistant burning mouth syndrome: a controlled study. Journal of Oral Pathology and Medicine 24:213–215

Casas J M, Beemsterboer P, Clark G T 1982 A comparison of stress-reduction counselling and contingent nocturnal EMG feedback for the treatment of bruxism. Behaviour Research and Therapy 20(1):9–15

Cohen R S 1995 Subjective reports on the effects of MDMA ('Ecstasy') experience in humans. Progress in Neuro Psychopharmacology and Biological Psychiatry 19(7):1137–1145

Cunningham S J, Bryant C J, Manisali M, Hunt N P, Feinmann C 1996 Dysmorphophobia: recent developments of interest to the maxillofacial surgeon. British Journal of Oral and Maxillofacial Surgery 34:368–374

Enoch D, Jagger R 1994 Psychiatric disorders in dental practice. Oxford: Wright

Fischer W F, O'Toole E T 1993 Personality characteristics of chronic bruxers. Behavioural Medicine 19(2):82–86

Fitzgerald K, Healy D 1995 Dystonias and dyskinesias of the jaw associated with the use of SSRIs. Human Psychopharmacology Clinical and Experimental, 10(3):215–219

Funch D, Gale E 1984 Biofeedback and relaxation therapy for chronic temporomandibular joint pain: predicting successful outcomes. Journal of Consulting and Clinical Psychology 52(6):928–935

Garro L 1994 Narrative representations of chronic illness experience: Cultural models of illness, mind, and body in stories concerning the temporomandibular joint (TMJ). Social Science and Medicine 38(6):775–788

Green R M, Humphris G M, Lindsay S J E, Mellor A, Millar K, Sidebotham B 1997 Minor psychiatric morbidity, pain and fear in patients in general dental practice. Community Dentistry and Oral Epidemiology 25:187–188

Humphris G M, Healey T, Howell R, Cawood J 1995 The psychological impact of implant-retained mandibular protheses: a cross-sectional study. International Journal of Maxillofacial Implants 10:437–444

Humphris G M, Longman L P, Field E A 1996 Cognitive behavioural therapy with two cases of Burning Mouth Syndrome. British Dental Journal 181:204–208

Kells B E, Kime D L, Kennedy J G, Freeman R 1996 Dysmorphophobia: a case successfully treated using a multidisciplinary approach. Dental Update (December) 402–403

Kent G, Johns R 1993 Psychological effects of permanently implanted false teeth: a two-year follow-up and comparison with dentate patients. Psychology and Health 8:213–222

Lester D 1997 Suicide. In: Baum A, Newman S, Weinman J, West R, McManus C (eds.) Cambridge Handbook of Psychology, Health and Medicine (pp. 602–603). Cambridge: Cambridge University Press

Milosevic A, Slade P D 1989. The orodental status of anorexics and bulimics. British Dental Journal 167:66–70

Moore R, Brodsgard I, Birn H 1991 Manifestations, acquisition and diagnostic categories of dental fear in a self-referred population. Behaviour Research and Therapy 29:51–60

Morris S, Benjamin S, Gray R, Bennett D 1997 Physical, psychiatric and social characteristics of the temporomandibular disorder pain dysfunction syndrome: the relationship of mental disorders to presentation. British Dental Journal 182:255–260

Morse D R 1982 Stress and bruxism: a critical review and report of cases. Journal of Human Stress 8(1):43–54

Mott A E, Grushka M, Sessle B J 1993 Diagnosis and management of taste disorders and Burning Mouth Syndrome. Dental Clinics of North America 37(1):33–71

Rosen J C, Reiter J, Orosan P 1995 Cognitive-behavioural body image therapy for Body Dysmorphic Disorder. Journal of Consulting and Clinical Psychology 63:263–269

Schuurs A H B 1988 Community Dentistry and Oral Epidemiology 16:274–277

van der Laan G , Duinkerke A, Luteijn F, van der Poel A 1988 Role of psychological and social variables in TMJ pain dysfunction syndrome (PDS) symptoms. Community Dentistry and Oral Epidemiology 16:274–277

Ware J C, Rugh J D 1988 Destructive bruxism: Sleep stage relationship. Sleep 11(2):172–181

10

Health education and health promotion

Case 10a Prevention in the practice

At a practice in the north-west of England the principal dentist was keen to encourage patients who smoke tobacco to quit the habit. The programme to be introduced into the practice would be evaluated by the principal examining the practice records every year to see if the percentage of patients who smoked had reduced. The intention was for the dentist to discuss with the patient the hazards to general health of continuing to smoke, and then to provide dental examples of how smoking prevents natural healing processes, making some treatments such as periodontal surgery unsuccessful and therefore contraindicated. The patient was to be persuaded to quit smoking on the basis that it was a risk to gingival health and to the soft tissues of the mouth such as the tongue and the insides of cheek and lips. The dental receptionists were given the task of asking the patients whether they smoked and this information would be passed over to the dentist, with the notes, who would then check what dental symptoms patients may have experienced. Unfortunately, patients took exception to being asked by a receptionist about their smoking behaviour. It seemed that attenders at the surgery had expected questions about smoking to come from the dentist and not from other members of the practice team. Patients felt that smoking behaviour was sensitive information.

This case scenario demonstrates some introductory points to note when embarking on a health promotion or education programme:

- A health problem is identified.
- The problem must be closely linked to behaviour or actions (of individuals, groups of people or those who are opinion formers such as local councillors, voluntary service organisers etc.).
- A target group is selected from available information such as health assessment surveys.
- The programme requires preparation of materials, training, piloting and an evaluation system to be designed.

The promotion of tobacco cessation in general dental practice is receiving attention from health promoters. Dental practice provides an opportunity to reach members of the public who may attend a dentist regularly, but receive little advice and support sufficient for individual smokers to consider changing their health behaviour. The methods employed have to be sensitively planned and implemented. The case above shows that staff need specific training and the programme requires a pilot phase to check that the approach is acceptable to patients. The aim of this chapter is to give definitions of health education and promotion and provide examples of how different approaches from individual to group interventions can be designed, implemented and evaluated.

Health education

The objective for all chairside dental health education should 'foster negotiation and collaboration with dental practitioners so that patients might be helped to make informed choices' (Sheiham & Croucher 1994). A wider definition is required to include activities not only in the dental practice but also in schools, the workplace, shopping and community areas. Definitions abound and this is an indication that health education as a field, and an activity, has been changing and developing over the years. One definition that focuses on health-related behaviour (that is, the behaviour may not be seen by the individual as necessarily enhancing health) and in addition concentrates on learning processes is as follows: 'any planned combination of learning experiences designed to predispose, enable, and reinforce voluntary behaviour conducive to health, in individuals, groups, or communities.' (Frazier 1992)

Health promotion

Health promotion however includes a far wider range of activities and is characterised by a combination of educational, organisational, economic and environmental supports for improving health through behaviour change (Cohen 1990). It has been defined (in a WHO workshop in June 1984) as 'the process of enabling individuals and communities to increase control over the determinants of health and thereby improve their health'. Features that have been highlighted are detailed below:

- A structure of principles focusing explicitly on oral disease prevention (Levine 1996).
- Public health programmes concerning the use of fluoride (e.g. toothpastes, fluoride supplements, mouth rinse programmes, water or milk fluoridation, and mass advertising of fluoride additives in toothpastes).
- Regular representative population surveys of dental health (e.g. the OPCS Adult and Child Dental Health Surveys of the UK).
- Advice sought by government from the dental organisations and bodies involved in public health.
- A commissioned research endeavour which encourages prevention and values the inclusion

of behavioural and social sciences (e.g. The UK NHS Research and Development Programme in Primary Dental Care which includes oral health promotion as one of its priority areas).

Health promotion is regarded by many authorities as including a healthy public health policy with an emphasis on a reduction of inequalities, multi-sectoral collaboration and community actions which rely on self-empowerment (Tones 1991). A belief in the ability of the self to achieve certain outcomes, known as self-efficacy belief, is an essential component for individuals acquiring a sense of empowerment. Health promotion programmes include references to lifestyle changes, personal development and the making of healthy choices (as opposed to focussing on a single prescribed behaviour) that are considered to foster empowerment. Additions to the empowerment cause include assisting community action and encouraging learning among communities about public health. Community action is therefore strengthened to improve health and thus encourage resources to be channelled into programmes that have been self-selected. These local actions and changing resource streams are often controversial and stimulate strongly held opinions. Political, ethical and moral dilemmas are often raised. Unfortunately, the term empowerment in this context has been overused and has lost some of its original significance. The empowerment principle is, however, an important one. Health promotion therefore places greater emphasis on planning compared with health education, and lays more emphasis upon legislative controls and sanctions, matched to local needs, as identified by community members (Milio 1986).

PLANNING

The importance of planning is highlighted in the Precede-Proceed model that lists five stages of planning which refer to making a detailed diagnosis (Green & Kreuter 1991). The first two stages (of the five stage 'precede' phase) include diagnosis from a social and epidemiological view. In other words the planner is attempting to understand the nature of the health difficulties of the group or community (epidemiological) and to what extent health is regarded as vital to quality of life, taking a broad set of views (social). An analysis of behaviour and how the environment impinges on health is the next stage in the diagnostic procedure. Stage four concentrates on the three factors (predisposing, enabling and reinforcing) which influence voluntary behaviour raised by Frazier in the definition cited already. The final diagnostic stage (administration and policy) looks carefully at the possibilities of adopting health education strategies and checks the regulatory and administrative structures. The 'proceed' phase includes four more stages, the first of which may be summarised as implementation of the health promotion activity and three further stages that focus on evaluation of the process, impact and outcome. See later in this chapter for an example of the 'proceed' arm of this planning model.

Whereas attention on health promotion developed in the 1970s with the World Health Organisation (WHO) publishing statements such as Health For All by the Year 2000 and a document on concepts and principles in the early 80s (WHO 1984), dental health education (which is subsumed under health promotion as a means of achieving health gains) began earlier. Since the 1920s four changes have taken place in dental health education (Towner 1993) and may be identified as:

1. A move towards participation by the public to improve learning experiences.
2. The inclusion of other disciplines has increased to help improve good practice and develop sophisticated programmes.
3. Dental health education has shifted to greater specificity of target groups.
4. There is less focus on increasing information to children.

Table 10.1

The Precede-Proceed Model

Phase Step		Description	Planning arm
1	Social	Identify health goals of target group	Precede
2	Epidemiological	Determine health problems	Precede
3	Behaviour and environment	Analyse behaviour and detect environmental influences	Precede
4	Education and organisation	Establish factors that will influence behaviour change	Precede
5	Administration and policy	Overcome barriers to introduce educational programme	Precede
6	IMPLEMENTATION	Redesign programme if difficulties are sufficient to demand it	Proceed
7	Process evaluation	Educational targets are examined	Proceed
8	Impact evaluation	Behavioural changes are assessed	Proceed
9	Outcome evaluation	Health outcome measures analysed for proximity to health goal	Proceed

Understanding health behaviour

Traditional health education has focused upon professionals who provide relevant information that increases knowledge which in turn changes attitudes and leads to improvements in health behaviour. Known as the K-A-B model (Knowledge-Attitudes-Behaviour), this model is now understood to be simplistic (Fig. 10.1). The link between the level of knowledge an individual possesses about a dental disease, such as caries, and their attitude towards it may not necessarily correspond. A person may know that sugar encourages caries but his attitude to caries may be neutral as he is aware that the decay can be treated at the dentist by filling material. The individual may even regard the newer white filling materials as more attractive than the original stained enamel. Similarly, the association between attitudes and behaviour may be weak. For instance, the person who recounts a positive view to attending the dentist may not take the steps necessary to make a visit. The steps required may include contacting a dental surgery to arrange an appointment, finding a convenient time and travelling to the surgery.

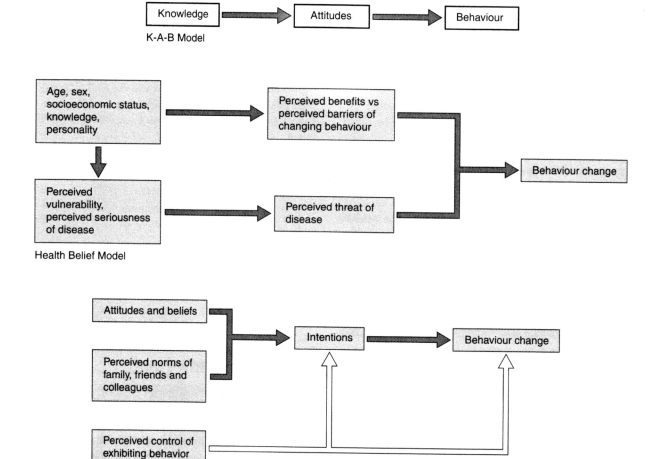

Fig. 10.1 Explaining health behaviours: three models. (In theory of Reasoned Actions shaded arrows; Theory of Planned Behaviour = shaded and clear arrows.)

Any one of these steps may not be fulfilled. A further example would be the potential patient who may not be able to take time off work to make a checkup visit. This case would be an example of external social factors impinging on the hypothesised relationship between attitudes and behaviour.

From these simple examples the K-A-B model can be shown to be limited and relatively unsophisticated. Two further points need to be raised. First, the direction of causation of knowledge influencing attitudes and, in turn, attitudes affecting behaviour is not automatic. There are many instances where causation is the reverse of that hypothesised. Children may be effectively taught to brush their teeth well by

following a simple demonstration (modelling). This is opposed to lengthy lessons improving their level of knowledge concerning toothbrushing. Appropriate knowledge and attitudes towards this behaviour may follow at a later stage. For many children, toothbrushing becomes a routine associated with washing the face and hands and brushing of hair (that is, grooming) and is less based upon a closely reasoned inspection of the purpose of the healthcare behaviour. Secondly, children may already know a great deal about toothbrushing and have positive attitudes. The influence of incidental information exchange through advertisements, magazines and the Internet (e-zines, health forums, etc.) should make dental health professionals consider carefully what additional facts would be helpful for their patients to receive.

A study to encourage improved oral hygiene procedures in adolescents by showing a 20-minute film found that knowledge levels increased by up to 40% but marginal effects were demonstrated on assessed attitudes and behaviour (ter Horst & Hoogstraten 1989). The authors concluded that a more extensive intervention was required to change the outcome behaviour. A further study attempting to show a positive relationship between knowledge about oral hygiene practices and behaviour (that is, utilisation of dental services over the previous five-year period) found no association (Bader et al. 1990). The investigators also assessed six periodontal condition measures (for example, plaque, gingivitis and calculus indexes). When the effects of age, gender, race and different practices were removed the association between knowledge and periodontal condition (i.e. the outcome measure) was not significant. The fact that the participants in the survey were regular attenders, with a low prevalence of disease, probably reduced the likelihood of demonstrating the expected relationship, as they may have been a uniform type of patient.

Social scientists have had mixed success in demonstrating a strong relationship between attitudes and behaviour. It is important to recognise that predicting health behaviour is far from straightforward. There are a large number of factors involved in establishing consistency between opinions held by a group of individuals and their behaviour. These factors will include, for example, the specificity and time frame of the attitudes being assessed, so that low associations between general attitudes and a single instance of a behaviour are observed (for example, attitudes towards dentists and relating these to whether a visit had been made to the dentist in the past six months). Those with positive views towards dentists may not have visited because they have a low perception of treatment need. This would be an example of not assessing the relevant attitude or belief. Further development of mechanisms and models of human social behaviour and reasoning are required to help explain health behaviour. The number of factors now known to be of relevance in understanding an individual's dental health

behaviour is great and requires a framework to study the relationships in some depth. This framework is sometimes referred to as a model. Some explanation of the underlying constructs – whether they are psychological or sociological in nature – and presenting these in a structured and coherent way will help develop the clinician's understanding further: interventions and assistance will therefore be more successful.

It is recognised that encouraging individuals to change their behaviour with respect to health is a considerable challenge. The endeavour to assist change attracts wide and enthusiastic interest. Dental personnel can, however, become cynical of educational packages which appear not to deliver the expected goals. Alternatively, a member of staff may design his own approach but finds that success is usually mixed at best. This section will examine some of the models that have been applied to understanding dental health behaviour.

The first important point is awareness of the actual behaviour which the health educator is attempting to explain and change. Table 10.2 shows that there are a substantial number of behaviours that could be classed as 'dental health behaviours'. Evidence is accumulating that each behaviour has its own sets of determinants. In other words, each behaviour will have its own unique set of factors that will assist the behaviour being conducted or alternatively prevent it from occurring. As an example, it is important to understand what promotes flossing: the introduction of free samples or instructing how to use floss may be effective in establishing the behaviour. These interventions may help to get over the barriers perceived by those who do not floss. People may say, for instance, that they do not know what packaging floss is sold in, and therefore can't recognise the product in the shops. Alternatively, they may complain that they do not have the manual dexterity to manage floss in their mouths. This belief may not be based on previous attempts but is given as justification for not using floss regularly. An offer of training in the use of floss by the hygienist may remove a block to the behaviour being adopted. Therefore a second point is that attempts to find a general attitude, belief or other psychological construct possessed by individuals that efficiently predicts a certain dental health behaviour have been elusive.

Table 10.2		

List of dental health behaviours and method of quantification

Behaviour	Specific	Measure (examples)
Visit to the dentist	•For checkup •When a symptom is experienced (e.g. toothache)	•Frequency per annum •Duration since last visit (ditto above)
Visit to the hygienist	•For prophylaxis and oral hygiene instruction	•Frequency per annum •Duration since last visit
Toothbrushing	•Hand •Electric	•Frequency per day •Duration •Time spent in each quadrant of the mouth (ditto above)
Toothpicks/ wooden sticks	•Interdental plaque removal	•Frequency per week
Floss	•Interdental plaque removal	•Frequency per week
Fluoride mouthwash	•Non-antiseptic fluoride concentrate •Antibacterial agent with fluoride additive	•Frequency per week (ditto above)
Snack eating	•With sugar •Non-sugar foods	•Frequency per week •Total grams ingested (ditto above)
Carbonated drinks	•With sugar •With sugar substitute or non-sugar	•Frequency per week •Total amount ingested (ditto above)

Social factors assist in identifying groups of people who may be likely – or not – to exhibit a certain health behaviour. Attempts to explain individual practices on this basis are not, however, successful. This situation may appear disheartening, but it does illustrate that trying to design an overall educational approach to be accepted by a wide population about general health matters is probably wasted effort. The complexity of trying to understand human behaviour gives the field its great attraction for many practitioners, health personnel and researchers. The implication of achieving a limited success in understanding dental health behaviour is that specific measures are required to be tailored to each target group selected. Approaches to some of the ways that have been formulated to understand health behaviour are covered briefly.

Health belief model

One of the most widely quoted models is the Health Belief Model (HBM) which has been applied in various guises since the late 1960s and early 1970s to the field of dental health. Some of these early studies in predicting dental attendance showed that if an individual believed that they were susceptible to dental caries, believed that caries would be serious if they contracted the disease, and that the benefits of visiting the dentist would be favourable then there was a greater likelihood that dental visiting will have occurred. It has been cited that over 7000 articles have already been published (not necessarily on dentistry alone) in the 1990s. The small study by Barker (43 adults took part) using the HBM to explain patient compliance with preventive dental advice from a teaching hospital showed that susceptibility and a belief in the benefit of the health behaviour were important aids in predicting future behaviour (Barker 1994). The comparatively small sample size and limited duration between assessment of beliefs and the enquiry into the actual behaviour exhibited makes the ability to generalise this result limited.

Another study, this time encouraging school age children to sign into a school-supervised fluoride additive scheme by attempting to actively change the children's health beliefs in the direction indicated by the HBM (that is, providing presentations that stated that the students were prone to caries and that there are some possibly serious consequences for them) found little evidence that changing health beliefs in the specified direction had any effect on enrolment into the programme (Weisenberg, Kegeles & Lund 1980). This study was important because the experimental design was sophisticated, using control groups and collecting data over a reasonable time span (referred to as a prospective study). Additional constructs have been included in a reformulated HBM, namely cues for action (for example, a spouse encouraging a partner to visit the dentist for a checkup) and health motivation. Even with the modifications to the HBM, it does suffer from the following drawbacks:

1. A strong emphasis on the disease rather than the behaviour which it tries to predict (almost as an afterthought in some cases).

2. It ignores the fact that people are not adding machines and that their beliefs are not neatly boxed up ready to be taped and a calculation run and accessed which has a direct line to triggering a behaviour. Behaviour is shaped by social forces and personal factors such as emotions and not solely by an economic appraisal of the pros and cons.

3. The HBM does not infer how the various components act together or separately on the behavioural targets, e.g. toothbrushing (Sheeran & Abraham 1995).

In its favour however is the fact that the HBM model uses psychological constructs that appeal to common sense (Conner & Norman 1995) and is often a good starting point for developing a framework of understanding a dental health activity (Eiser 1997). To demonstrate how aspects of the model can be very helpful in assisting clinical management of a patient was shown by a case report that found that mistaken health beliefs were responsible for severe ulceration of the gingiva (Pearlman 1994). The patient believed that strong scrubbing with his toothbrush would help to make his gums bleed, and he regarded bleeding gums as a sign that he was brushing well. Unfortunately he had misconstrued the message and believed that bleeding gums were only an indicator initially of a rigorous oral hygiene campaign. This health belief however is not part of the HBM but rather a feature of another model, the Theory of Reasoned Action (TRA). The TRA concentrates on how the behaviour is expected to occur from a set of beliefs and attitudes about the behaviour in question *rather than the emphasis on disease*. The patient's beliefs about the behaviour were changed by informing him that over-enthusiastic brushing would prove damaging to the gums. He was taught to brush properly after a period of completely stopping toothbrushing. He used an antiseptic mouthwash and had methods of non-traumatic toothbrushing explained. Future months cleared the initial ulceration and in the longer term his gingival health was good.

Theory of reasoned action

The Theory of Reasoned Action (TRA) presents a model to predict behaviour which utilises the beliefs held by individuals. There are however important differences and additions over the HBM. First, the TRA includes only beliefs about an intended behaviour (for example, 'How strongly do you believe that not taking sugar in your hot drinks will prevent you from getting tooth decay?') as opposed to concentrating on beliefs about disease alone. Second, an evaluation of the outcome of the behaviour is introduced (e.g. 'How important is it to you that if you stop taking sugar in hot drinks it will help prevent tooth decay?'). Fishbein and Ajzen (1980) predict an individual's attitude by multiplying the belief by the outcome evaluation: according to the TRA model, this will assist in estimating behavioural intention. Third, an important element ignored by the HBM is the inclusion of an individual's beliefs about what others may think of them performing the health action (or not performing the action). Behaviour is often shaped and promoted by other people (Fig. 10.1). These people are sometimes referred to as normative referents. A key component of the TRA is to determine who the individual believes has an influence on them with respect to the behaviour and how strong this influence is.

A recent example of the application of the TRA to dental health behaviour is a study with adolescents attempting to understand the attitudes and normative referents to sugar consumption in hot drinks such as tea and coffee (Freeman & Sheiham 1997). An essential stage in the application of this model is the careful interviewing of the target group to identify their key beliefs and referents. These authors found two distinct behaviours that required different beliefs to explain each of them. They found that the inclusion or exclusion of sugar in hot drinks was a helpful distinction to make: the predictors for including sugar were attitudes and also other related dental health behaviours such as regularity of dental attendance and toothbrushing. Interestingly the predictor for excluding sugar from hot drinks was dental attendance and dental health knowledge. In summary, this study found that the conceptual structure of the TRA was valuable as it required the investigators to inspect closely the behaviour they were trying to predict: they found also that there were really two distinct aspects of behaviour that could be analysed and therefore required separate analysis. Further, by interviewing members of the target group the beliefs that are relevant to the individuals themselves are identified rather than some preselected beliefs that are likely to be a reflection of the researchers' beliefs. Finally, prediction of intentions to use, or stop, sugar consumption in tea and coffee, included some aspects of the TRA but also other behaviours. For instance, using sugar was predicted by individuals reporting that they attended the dentist regularly whereas attempts to stop using sugar were explained by a record of infrequent dental attendance. The extent that some health behaviours may be associated is an important issue raised later in the chapter. The same cautionary remark made concerning the HBM also applies to this example study. Namely, the issue of using cross-sectional data (that is, a collection of questionnaire responses at a single point in time) to demonstrate a dynamic system of apparent change in beliefs, attitudes and behaviour is relevant. Studies which follow a cohort of participants over time (a longitudinal study) will produce greater understanding of what determines health behaviour and what methods can be applied to encourage behavioural change.

The TRA has been extended to include a further explanatory construct. The degree that health-related behaviours can be performed will be a function of how much the individual believes that the behaviour will occur and the extent that they personally exert any control over the behaviour. For example, predicting the dental checkup frequency of secondary school children would be seriously deficient unless some account was taken of the level of control that children considered they had to initiate or refuse attending the dentist. This model has been named the Theory of Planned Behaviour (Fig. 10.1) and has been shown, in comparison with the TRA, to improve explanation of the behaviour under scrutiny (Ajzen 1991). With all of the above models, HBM, TRA and TPB, it can be seen that some thought processing by the individual takes place to perform a particular health-related behaviour. The health promoter will

gain in taking time and trouble to understand this processing in order to design programmes which may influence individual's thinking.

Transtheoretical model of change

As described already, systematic attempts to understand health-directed and health-related behaviours have relied principally on single stage models. Other models, not presented here for reasons of space, demonstrate this same feature: that is, no distinction is made as to what beliefs, attitudes or social pressures are required and in what order before a change in behaviour can be expected. A notable exception is the transtheoretical model of change put forward to explain addictive behaviours. The most well known application is the prediction of tobacco smoking (Prochaska & DiClemente 1984). This is a five-stage model and at each of the five stages certain processes are required. The five stages of change – illustrated by the example of smoking (in brackets) – are:

1. Pre-contemplation (not aware that smoking is a problem and therefore has no intention to stop).
2. Contemplation (the smoker is starting to consider the pros and cons of smoking but has not firmly stated any intention to quit).
3. Preparation (an intention to quit is made and plans are made to attempt to give up smoking).
4. Action (an active attempt to stop smoking is in evidence).
5. Maintenance (after a period of time – six months – the smoker attempts to prevent a relapse and takes on the new role of abstainer).

The processes at each stage are discrete activities and these are listed in Table 10.3. For example consciousness raising is a process that includes attempts to increase awareness of own views and responses plus obtaining new information about the focused behaviour. The model expects the individual to move in a positive direction from pre-contemplator to maintainer. Empirical evidence suggests that people move at different rates through the stages, occasionally reverting back a stage, or sticking at a stage for a long period without further progression. In reality, the way people change their behaviour is not as neatly followed as the model suggests, although the model does enjoy a good deal of support.

The helpfulness of this approach may be summarised as follows:

- It alerts the health educator to the possible difficulties in achieving behavioural change. That is, the individual has to undergo a number of separate stages before success is achieved. A move to the next stage is regarded as positive.
- There is potential both for moving forwards or remaining static. In addition, although this is not stated explicitly in the model but rather inferred from empirical observation, the

individual can revert back a stage: the contemplator may for example revert back to being a pre-contemplator. Another example would be the person who instigates action to change but may be unable to sustain the behaviour and return to a previous stage.

Evidence from the tobacco cessation field shows that before successful maintenance is achieved in quitting smoking the average smoker revolves around the whole five-stage cycle on three occasions. The average length of time to arrive at maintenance from the stage of pre-contemplation is around five years. This should both encourage and discourage potential health promoters. The evidence for behavioural change is positive in that it can and does occur, but the difficulties encountered by individuals are far greater than many health professionals have sometimes been willing to accept. The fact that people can proceed through a cycle of stages perhaps relapsing a number of times before reaching a sustained level of behavioural change should demonstrate to healthcare workers that a single one-off programme is of limited value and will only assist perhaps a small proportion of people, and this small group are probably in the throes of taking action already. Sustained effort over time and recognising that the target group will be at different stages of behavioural change will assist a more sensitive programme development with longer term goals. A difficulty of this stage-approach model is that it still does not tell us how or why people move from one stage to another. The field of motivational study is sometimes called upon to help answer these questions.

MOTIVATION

Practitioners and healthcare workers are keen to determine how to 'motivate' their patients or client group. Typically motivators may rely on making appeals to fear or highlighting the benefits of change. Fear appeals are based upon frightening the patient to adopt a particular behaviour, whereas indicating the advantages of a recommended action relies on less ethically questionable tactics. Simply giving very clear instructions has also been advocated as an aid to changing behaviour. Interventions designed for school oral

---

Table 10.3

Processes of change described by the transtheoretical model and at what stage the process is believed to occur (some processes overlap two stages)

Model stage	Process	Description of process
C	Consciousness-raising	Increase in self-awareness about the target behaviour.
C,A	Self-evaluation	Change of own emotional and cognitive response to the relevant behaviour.
A	Self-liberation	Recognition that change will produce a release of old constraints.
A	Helping relationship	Accepting assistance from others to make a change.
A	Reinforcement management	Acceptance of rewards from self and others for changing behaviour.
A,M	Counter-conditioning	Substitute alternative behaviours, e.g. eating satisfying non-sugar snacks instead of sweets and biscuits.
A,M	Stimulus control	Avoiding situations and places where signals of problem behaviour would previously have helped to trigger a response, or alternatively placing reminders to promote a behaviour, e.g. note stuck on bathroom mirror to floss.

Key to stages: C: Contemplation; A: Action; M: Maintenance

hygiene programmes with a sophisticated evaluation system (repeated dental plaque assessments) found that the persuasive message which stressed the benefits were more likely to produce an improvement in outcome. These results were not straightforward due to some evidence showing that at extended follow-up 'scare tactics' indicated the best result. The difficulty is being aware of what will motivate a certain individual. From the previous discussion above the possibility of healthcare personnel guessing the appropriate motivator for an individual or a group is unlikely. A more behavioural approach that adopts first principles is recommended, as referred to in Chapter 4. Behaviour once performed has consequences which are either favourable or unfavourable. If favourable then the likelihood of behaviour being repeated is increased. The behaviour is regarded as having been positively rewarded. Alternatively, unfavourable consequences will result in behaviour being less likely to be performed, a process known as extinction. Please note that negative reinforcement is a case where some behaviour is encouraged to prevent a negative consequence e.g. an adult with exposed dentine choosing warm milk to drink, as opposed to an ice-cool beverage, thereby avoiding discomfort.

There are many examples of using positive reinforcement to increase the likelihood of behavioural change. When two groups of patients were offered oral hygiene programmes and one group was offered a 25% reduction in cost if their plaque scores were reduced it was found that an immediate improvement was observed which was maintained for six months (Iwata & Becksford 1981). In addition there has been a study of rural, low-income families in the USA who were encouraged to have dental checkups by a prompting letter and a returnable monetary voucher. The interesting finding from this study was that the one-off offer of a voucher promoted subsequent follow-up visits even though no further monetary assistance was provided (Reiss, Piotrowski & Bailey 1976). These studies demonstrated that when effective reinforcers are identified, behaviour will change. A recent review (of 11 studies: two dental, nine medical) has highlighted the possible benefits of enhancing patient compliance through financial incentives (Giuffrida & Torgerson 1997). Although financial reinforcement may appear to be an obvious 'motivator' consider that the maintenance of behaviour in the Iwata and Becksford and Reiss studies (continued low plaque levels or increased frequency of regular checkups) was not dependent on further monetary rewards. The implication for these and other similar studies of this type is that the participants are acting on an effective reinforcement. Examples of other reinforcers include receipt of praise from staff, meeting friends or acquaintances at the health centre, acquiring useful information, receiving advice or offers of help in associated areas of concern, feeling part of a group and satisfying a social pressure to belong to a certain group (Weinstein et al. 1996). When other reinforcers substitute for an original reinforcer this is known as secondary reinforcement. It is likely that the maintenance of behaviour shown in the Reiss study is an example of secondary reinforcers such as warmth of welcome, praise for visiting, sense of belonging etc., that the dental team were able to impart to the visiting families.

An important concept derived from the transtheoretical model of change is 'readiness to change' (Rollnick, Kinnersky & Stott 1993). Attempts to ascertain the willingness of individuals to make a change in their behaviour (whether it is to modify or adopt a new health-related behaviour) is regarded as vital so as not to waste resource (materials, staff time) and not to 'inoculate' the individual. If techniques are applied to patients who are not keen to change their behaviour then the approach will lose its novelty and even increase resistance to adoption or adherence to a recommendation.

SELF-ASSESSMENT

Perception of need for treatment is a similar concept to readiness to change. The latter explicitly refers to behavioural change whereas perception is a psychological belief. However, it is helpful in assisting individuals to consider their perception of, for example, disease level or impairment. This may be achieved by encouraging self-assessment. The effectiveness as determined by a reduction in gingival bleeding sites of two types of self-assessment over a two-year period was shown in

14–15 year olds (Nowjack-Raymer et al. 1995). The trial was school-based and involved some minimal training from hygienists, and the use of written manuals. The two types of assessment included the teenager either identifying the number of bleeding points or locating the number of areas of plaque in the mouth with the aid of disclosing tablets. Some evidence exists to show that adolescents can indeed assess sufficiently well enough for monitoring gingival health (Kallio & Murtomaa 1997).

EMPOWERMENT

Approaches that involve self-assessment have merit as they assist individuals themselves to identify a potential problem for which they can seek treatment. Such methods satisfy the concept of enabling individuals to select and make their own choices over their health rather than respond somewhat automatically to advice from a specialist campaign which is not integrated and may only be present for a short period of time. This issue of 'empowerment', as mentioned earlier in this chapter, is important in the health promotion field as it helps to restore a balance in favour of the non-specialist individual who is paradoxically a specialist and expert about his own body, desires, responsibilities and concerns. This balancing of the various agendas held by the health specialist and by members of the public is satisfied by a process of negotiation, required to identify the most appropriate path in achieving the desired outcome for both parties. It should be recognised that negotiations do not always succeed and an extension in time may be required before a new bargaining position can be encountered and agreed.

EVALUATION

Health education programmes are a challenge to evaluate. But while there are many examples of poor evaluations, conducting some form of evaluation should be considered essential when introducing a programme. The temptation to utilise every available portion of resource to the educational intervention so as to impart the maximum effect should be avoided. Poor evalua-

tion may compromise the message/intervention that is introduced as the methodology was so poor that even a strong effect from the programme would have been missed or improperly assessed. Evaluation should focus on three aspects which follow Green's Precede-Proceed model, namely process, impact and outcome.

Case 10b The importance of planning for successful evaluation

A programme designed by a Health Authority community dental service to influence adolescents' snacking behaviour was introduced into a number of schools in a locality that showed high levels of caries in this age group. The adolescents were informed about the harmful effects certain foods may have on teeth and gums. The process measures included the number of times that the message was repeated in the classroom, the length of time that the dental health educator spent in each class explaining the project, and the willingness of teachers to include dental-related topics in the classwork. The impact measures included assessments of dental knowledge, especially focused on the influence of frequent sugar intake on plaque formation, and self-reports of diet diaries. The outcome measure included the sales of sugary snacks from the school shop. It was found that there was no change in the outcome measure with the introduction of the programme. The conclusion was not that the programme had failed but rather that the outcome measure had not been sensitive enough. Further questioning of some of the children from one school revealed evidence that fewer visits were made to local shops. The purchasing of snacks outside the school was not included in the outcome measure. The process and impact measures were consulted to determine if the initial objectives of the intervention were met. Knowledge of snack eating affecting dental health (an impact measure) showed a sharp improvement. It would be fair to assume that this improvement was caused by the class teaching. The diet diaries showed a very small decrease in sugar containing snacks and drinks, although the students were responsible for reporting their own behaviour and may have given favourable responses. Modification of the intervention may be required. A classroom teaching approach advocating the benefits to dental health from avoiding sugary snacks may not be sufficient to encourage young students to avoid sugar: a concentration on the reinforcers to be obtained from purchasing other foods instead of sugar-containing snacks would be appropriate. Hence, more attention spent on planning as mentioned at the start of the chapter would lead to greater success. Improvement of measures would also make the programme effects easier to interpret.

The fact that different reinforcers will appeal to different individuals in making behavioural changes explains why the effectiveness of various educational programmes do not differ markedly. The study by Lim is a good example of an evaluation of different modes of dental health education in the form of oral hygiene instruction with the exception that the study had not included a control group (Lim et al. 1996). No prophylaxis was performed during the study period, therefore the change in hygiene status could be attributed to the education received. The various modes which were presented to young adults working for a Hong Kong telephone company included: (1) personal instruction; (2) a self-instruction manual; (3) video; or (4) a combination of two or more of these modes of instruction. Two gingival health indices (plaque and gingival sulcus bleeding) were collected at baseline, two weeks, four months and at ten months. Reductions in the indices (mean %) were found at each follow-up period compared to baseline, although no differences were found between the various modes of instruction (as shown by comparison of percentage reduction from each of the randomised groups receiving a particular form of oral hygiene instruction). The lack of distinction between the modes of instruction tends to show that the method may not be the vital factor in gaining improvement in the health outcome measure – this was a function of the behaviour change, which was better plaque removal. Other explanations are available. The measurement of gingival condition and meeting the personnel on a regular basis for the checks to be performed may have contributed to the improved hygiene. There may have been some psychological gain in meeting with the investigation team during the study period which was responsible for the changes. The inclusion of two control groups would have assisted interpretation here. The first control group would not receive any instruction but simply be assessed at the same time points in the study period, while the second control group would be assessed at baseline and at the final follow-up point (i.e. ten months). If the measurement process had no influence on oral hygiene status then there should be no improvement in the indexes over time for both control groups. The first control group should show some positive changes during the study period, if repeated measures of oral hygiene impress the participants to increase this preventive behaviour. The outcome measures themselves may not have been sensitive enough to demonstrate differences, so that additional studies are required to replicate the study using somewhat more sophisticated measures. It can be seen that the interpretation of evaluative studies requires careful thought and attention to a myriad of factors. These are revisited again in Chapter 11 which focuses on research methods.

Barriers to change

The study by Lim did not investigate those participants who showed little or no change in oral hygiene. Extra information may be gleaned from studies of this nature to determine which individuals respond and those that do not. There may be some common features that help describe the category of persons that do not change their behaviour. Some caution has to be expressed with the identification of factors which may be considered as a barrier to change, as the categorical approach could introduce what is called 'victim blaming'. The non-responding group, sharing a particular feature, may be scapegoated for their failure to respond to a particular programme. Programme campaigners have to accept that their programme has unfortunately not identified the appropriate reinforcers that will encourage behavioural change in the non-responders.

An innovative Scottish study focusing on adolescents (15–17 years of age) sought to encourage the step of visiting the dentist by stressing the benefits of attendance, namely maintaining good facial appearance and providing a non-dental reinforcer or incentive (a discount voucher for a local fashion store). The campaign was successful but seemed to appeal to younger girls, who were intending to stay on at school and who were already regular attenders (Craven, Blinkhorn & Schou 1994). Of interest was the lack of a relationship between social class (measured by the ACORN system) and those who made a dental visit. The incentive scheme appealed widely across the sample of young people but was not successful with boys. Further analysis of results revealed a limited perception of need among those that did not respond. An attempt to reduce barriers, by bringing the surgery closer to the individual through the introduction of mobile units visiting the schools concerned, was advocated. In addition the authors encouraged a focus on younger adolescents. They remarked that over a third of the participants in the study were responsible for organising their own dental care, a finding that is consistent with other reports (Adekoya-Sofowora, Lee & Humphris 1996). The issue of trying to determine barriers to behavioural change and the highlighting of certain groups becomes a sensitive one if structural factors are implicated. This area has been analysed by Schou and colleagues, who have found in their Scottish campaigns that the influence of dental health education to the whole population does not seem to remove inequalities of dental health behaviour. The Lothian dental health campaign (Schou & Wight 1994) targeting five year old schoolchildren's oral hygiene and gingival health was found to have made a substantial overall impact on gingival health across the geographical area of the campaign, which included visits to local schools by community dental officers, encouraging teachers to take part and a home-care pack of information for parents including a toothbrush. However when the children from deprived areas were compared with children from more affluent areas it was found that the education campaign had provided very little benefit to the children from the deprived schools. Unfortunately the authors were not able to provide details of why the campaign was not influential in the deprived areas but recommended that health education efforts are designed and evaluated to take into account the appropriate needs of the different population groups.

Conditions necessary for behaviour change

Another approach in learning how to help people change their behaviour is to ask those who have succeeded already and understand the minimum conditions required for a change to occur. Some interesting results have emerged suggesting that six conditions are necessary:

1. People have to want to change. For people to change their behaviour it has to be self-initiated. Simple instructions, although helpful, will not in themselves generate a change.
2. The behaviour has to be salient. Events that impinge on individuals should highlight the behaviour as requiring their focus and attention: for example, local 'Smile Weeks' can often provide a stimulus in alerting people to consider their snack-eating behaviour.
3. The salience of the behaviour needs to be extended over time. Therefore simple interventions (lasting a short period) need to be backed up with a further extended programme. The introduction of legislation (local or national) or institutional regulation would assist the maintenance of behaviour change. For instance, a recommendation to remove sugary drinks from vending machines in educational establishments would reduce the likelihood of trainees (and their trainers) consuming harmful beverages.

4. The behaviour to be changed should not constitute a feature of the person's coping strategy. For example some people may chew gum which they use to relax in stressful situations. Chewing gum is also adopted in people with dry mouth syndrome and in some cases of chronic facial pain. It is difficult to advocate a ban on chewing gum in such instances. With the widespread introduction of sugarless gum (with sales now greater than the sugar variety) the chewing behaviour can be maintained with a switch to a sugarless brand.

5. The person's life must not be undergoing extensive change or uncertainty. People who are moving house, changing job, threatened with redundancy or some other unpredictable event will not be receptive to changing health behaviour.

6. The individual will require social support. For someone to make a change in their behaviour they will require reminders, praise and understanding on a fairly frequent basis. Family, including children, can act as a crucial support structure in maintaining behaviour change. Telephone helplines provide a readily accessible form of specialised assistance. QUIT, for example, is a charitable organisation specialising in the counselling of those who wish to stop smoking, and it has established expertise in the counselling of those from deprived communities.

Skills required for oral health promotion

The skills necessary to develop effective health promotion and education programmes are diverse. To start with, a knowledge of the disease processes and causative agents responsible for oral disease is important. Also important is a fundamental understanding of health needs assessment, community action planning (including the devising of coherent strategies for localities), the setting of goals, design of interventions, resources allocation and priority setting, and a knowledge of evaluation designs. The willingness to relinquish one's own involvement and encourage community members to take leadership, and communication skills with individuals, groups and local media are just some of the additional and varied skills that the professional serious about health promotion should exhibit (Watt & Fuller 1997). It should be clear that the single 'hero-innovator' approach of one person attempting to create a marked change in a community's health (whether it be dental or general health) is unlikely to succeed and therefore networks of personnel from health and other related disciplines (social workers, teachers, public health dentists and medics, town planners, social scientists) are recommended. The building of teams at a professional level with community participation in order to integrate oral health preventive activities into general health systems such as primary care has received attention under the name of 'teamwork' (Nowjack-Raymer 1995). However actual collaborative teams are difficult to find as the roles expected of the individuals concerned are not ones that are comfortable for many who might constitute such teams. The skills needed to assist a team to run effectively include:

- The ability to tolerate uncertainty.
- Sharing responsibility collectively.
- Compromising to allow decisions to be made.
- Turn-taking so that all members have a share in leading the team.
- Resources to aid development and support of the team.

Teams are often employed across a number of sectors (e.g. hospital and community health centres, social services and housing authorities) to institute health programmes. However, dental practices and clinics are gaining in size and many of the principles of team-working can also be applied within these groupings of staff. Clarity must exist in the responsibilities that are held for clinical matters and those for the health promoting activities. The responsibility for clinical decisions remains with the individual clinician. Implementation of programmes following the planning stages from such teams requires organisational skills, energy, diplomacy and persistence to successfully introduce such a campaign.

References

Adekoya-Sofowora C, Lee G, Humphris G 1996 Needs for dental information of adolescents from an inner city area of Liverpool. British Dental Journal 180:339–343

Ajzen I, Fishbein M 1980 Understanding attitudes and predicting social behaviour. Englewood Cliffs, NJ: Prentice Hall

Ajzen I 1991 The theory of planned behaviour. Organisational behaviour and human decision processes 50:179–211

Bader J, Rozier R, McFall W, Ramsey D 1990 Association of dental health knowledge with periodontal condition among regular patients. Community Dentistry and Oral Epidemiology 18:32–36

Barker T 1994 Role of health beliefs in patient compliance with preventive dental advice. Community Dentistry and Oral Epidemiology 22:327–330

Cohen L 1990 Promoting oral health: Guidelines for dental associations. International Dental Journal 40:79–102

Conner M, Norman P 1995 Predicting health behaviour. Buckingham: Open University Press

Craven R, Blinkhorn A, Schou L 1994 A campaign encouraging dental attendance among adolescents in Scotland: the barriers to behaviour change. Community Dental Health 11:131–134

Eiser R 1997 Attitudes and beliefs. In Baum A, Newman S, Weinman J, West R, McManus C (eds.) Cambridge Handbook of Psychology, Health and Medicine (pp. 3–7). Cambridge: Cambridge University Press

Frazier P 1992 Research on oral health education and promotion and social epidemiology. Journal of Public Health Dentistry 52:18–22

Freeman R, Sheiham A 1997 Understanding decision-making processes for sugar consumption in adolescence. Community Dentistry and Oral Epidemiology 25:228–232

Giuffrida A, Torgerson D 1997. Should we pay the patient? Review of financial incentives to enhance patient compliance. British Medical Journal 315:703–707

Green L, Kreuter M 1991 Health promotion planning: An educational and environmental approach. Mountain View, CA: Mayfield

Iwata B A, Becksford C M 1981 Behavioural research in preventive dentistry. Journal of Applied Behavioural Analysis 14:111–120

Kallio P, Murtomaa H 1997 Determinants of self-assessed gingival health among adolescents. Acta Odontologica Scandinavica 55:106–110

Levine R. 1996. The scientific basis of dental health education (4th edn.) London: Health Education Authority

Lim L, Davies W, Yuen K, Ma M 1996 Comparison of modes of oral hygiene instruction in improving gingival health. Journal of Clinical Periodontology 23:693–697

Milio N 1986 Promoting health through public policy. Ottawa: Canadian Public Health Association

Nowjack-Raymer R 1995 Teamwork in prevention: possibilities and barriers to integrating oral health into general health. Advances in Dental Research 9(2):100–105

Nowjack-Raymer R, Ainamo J, Suomi J, Kingman A, Driscoll W, Brown L 1995. Improved periodontal status through self-assessment: A 2-year longitudinal study in teenagers. Journal of Clinical Periodontology 22:603–608

Pearlman B 1994 A mistaken health belief resulting in gingival injury: a case report. Journal of Periodontology 65:284–286

Prochaska J, DiClemente C 1984 The transtheoretical approach: Crossing traditional boundaries. Homewood, IL: Irwin

Reiss M, Piotrowski W, Bailey J 1976 Behavioural community psychology: encouraging low-income patients to seek dental care for their children. Journal of Applied Behavioural Analysis 9:387–397

Rollnick S, Kinnersky P, Stott 1993. Methods of helping patients with behaviour change. British Medical Journal 307:188–190

Schou L, Wight C 1994 Does dental health education affect inequalities in dental health? Community Dental Health 11:97–100

Sheeran P, Abraham C 1995 The health belief model. In: Conner M, Norman P (eds.) Predicting health behaviour Buckingham: Open University Press

Sheiham A, Croucher R 1994 Current perspectives on improving chairside dental health education for adults. International Dental Journal 44:202–206

ter Horst G, Hoogstraten J 1989 Immediate and delayed effects of dental health education film on periodontal knowledge, attitudes, and reported behaviour of Dutch adolescents. Community Dentistry and Oral Epidemiology 17:183–186

Tones K 1991 Health promotion, empowerment and the psychology of control. Journal of the Institute of Health Education 29:17–26

Towner E 1993 The history of dental health education: a case study of Britain. In: Schou L, Blinkhorn A (eds.) Oral Health Promotion Oxford: Oxford University Press

Watt R, Fuller S 1997 Approaches in oral health promotion. In: Pine C (ed.), Community Oral Health Oxford: Wright

Weinstein R, Tosolin F, Ghilardi L, Zanardelli E 1996 Psychological intervention in patients with poor compliance. Journal of Clinical Periodontology 23:283–288

Weisenberg M, Kegeles S, Lund A 1980 Children's health beliefs and acceptance of a dental preventive activity. Journal of Health and Behaviour 21:59–74

WHO (1984). Health promotion: A discussion document on the concept and principles World Health Organisation Regional Office for Europe

Research in dental behavioural sciences

Identifying a topic for research

When asked to do some research to fulfil an assignment, the task can appear both exciting and daunting. How to progress with a project can, however, very quickly produce a general dislike for the whole organised area of enquiry unless some guidelines are followed. The traditions, technicalities and jargon that accompany much research endeavour may discourage even the most inquisitive and enthusiastic novice. This chapter aims to encourage you to persevere with such projects during your student career. Some of the procedures and decisions you need to appreciate in this chapter when embarking on your own projects are outlined. An understanding of how to conduct research will also help when appraising contacts with other health professionals who are keen to invite you to collaborate or when constructively criticising other people's published work. As an introduction this account urges you to become more conversant with research methods and to consider setting up studies of your own. Those

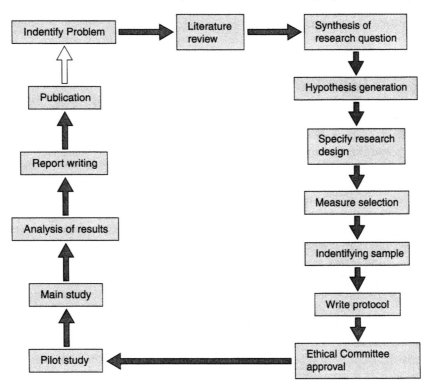

Fig 11.1 Process in conducting a research study.

healthcare workers who try to solve problems more formally in the workplace are those who are better informed and more open to alternative explanations for observed phenomena.

The selection of a problem for investigation may be determined by what is already known. However it can involve identifying issues which require further exploration. For the inexperienced clinician or new entrant to a profession or discipline it is advisable to seek the opinions of more senior staff. Original thinking may challenge traditional ideas and therefore other authorities should sometimes be consulted. There are a number of subject areas that social scientists in the dental health field have studied which may have been challenging, but were nonetheless important to study. Examples include investigating how dental students are socialised into becoming dentists, and a study of young people who take the drug Ecstasy and the influence of this on the erosion of their dentition. It is surprising that a great deal of research is conducted without a considered preparatory period. Fig. 11.1 shows the stage by stage process in conducting a research study. Constructing the question for study is an essential starting point: searching the literature is the next major hurdle.

Reviewing the literature

The modern literature search has changed out of all recognition to that of even a decade ago. The researcher of today has the benefit of electronic aids which can retrieve and filter through vast amounts of available written material. The abstract collections held on CD-ROMs which enable selection by key words such as scientific terms of interest or a particular author have transformed literature searching. The dental student will find the Medline and to some extent the Psyclit databases of abstracts a good place to start. A surprising number of articles do not find their way into these main collections and other services are needed. The Bath Information and Data Service (BIDS) is an online reference database which includes all references that a particular journal article has cited as well as abstracts. It is a powerful method of ensuring that a more comprehensive approach

is taken as the diligent reviewer will check the cited references for areas of interest. Searching the abstracts of higher degrees (dissertation abstracts) can provide an up-to-date assessment of a particular area about to be studied. Some flexibility of search terms is required and the assistance of the librarian can be helpful in improving inclusiveness of a search without retrieving a mass of redundant material. The role of systematic reviews of the literature has grown recently with the establishment in the medical and dental fields of the Cochcrane Collaboration. This commission reviews from volunteer researchers internationally and adds them to a bank which is open for inspection by interested parties. Guidelines in the form of a handbook have been issued and are (available on the World Wide Web – the URL for their handbook is: http://hiru.mcmaster.ca/cochrane/default.html). These guidelines assist in making decisions about suitable articles to include and offers a suitable weighting of studies to derive a coherent and generally acceptable framework for presenting key findings. Of course the rules of systematic reviewing are open to debate and no doubt will alter in time as views of what is considered appropriate scientific endeavour change.

Synthesis of the research question

The genesis of a research question is probably the most difficult task in conducting a successful project and many attempts are often required to hone and fine tune the wording. The student must seek supervision before arriving at the final written version. The importance of having an underlying theory should be apparent from the work already quoted in previous chapters. Much if not all of the studies referred to will have implicitly or explicitly stated a theory that assisted in the development of the research question. As already stated, some research projects are based on very little previous knowledge – other projects are linked very carefully to previous work in order that knowledge is acquired in a progressive and gradual fashion. On occasion replication of a study is warranted with an additional element included which the investigator has considered an alternative factor in explaining the published findings.

BOX 11.1   TYPES OF RESEARCH DESIGN

- Exploratory   Collect a number of variables through interview, questionnaire or observation and then test out a number of weakly composed hypotheses, often to follow up a 'hunch'.

- Experimental   Construct a study in which there are some strict controls on the variables you are interested in. Relies crucially on random allocation for most of these designs.

Clinical trial (CT)   Often regarded as the 'gold standard' design although limited to specific research questions, for example is one drug better than another?

Matched control   Similar to the CT although even more strictures are applied to the participants invited into the study.

- Descriptive   This is a design which relies on careful observation and description of events, behaviour etc. Used by the early scientists and still regarded as a central tool for hypothesis generation.

- Secondary analysis   More popular now that a methodology (meta-analysis) has been recognised to assist in the compilation of results from many studies. Meta-analysis has formal rules of how to combine the effects of an intervention from a number of previously published studies. Also includes re-analysis of interview transcripts.

- Single case design   Under-utilised design. The single individual acts as their own control over time where different interventions are applied and investigated.

- Observational   Highly technical procedures required to collate meaningful and often very illuminating data.

- Cross-sectional   Designs which provide a snapshot of an event or behaviour. They are relatively straightforward to implement.

- Longitudinal   Designs which follow a series of people, dental practices, etc. over time to assess change or causal processes. Complex and sophisticated to implement.

Specifying the study design

There is a huge variety of research designs (summarised in Box 11.1), each with their advantages and disadvantages. The design is chosen to optimise the chances of answering the research question, and there are two major categories of research used in the behavioural science area: qualitative and quantitative. As the nature of the term suggests, qualitative refers to a 'lifting of a veil' or 'unearthing' (terms employed by Blumer as cited by Hammersley 1996 p165) features of objects that have hitherto escaped researchers' ability to record or observe. Qualitative research is often erroneously regarded as working with words. Equally, quantitative research is frequently seen as dealing only with numbers, i.e. entities are assessed along some scale (see Table 11.1).

Traditionally, qualitative and quantitative studies have been portrayed as diametrically opposed

Table 11.1

Classification of scales from Nominal, Ordinal, Interval and Ratio (NOIR)

Scale	Description	Example
Nominal	A variable is expressed as categories with no order in terms of one category being greater or less than another category.	Gender is categorised as either female or male. Other nominal scales include various ethnic groupings, or types of dental practices such as urban, suburban or rural.
Ordinal	A scale that comprises at least two categories in which an order is reflected by degree. An ordinal scale is often regarded as a rating that can be ranked. There is an undisputed 'order' to the scale.	An attitude scale is commonly expressed as an ordinal scale. The degree of agreement can be expressed as a three-category scale ranging from disagree, neutral, agree.
Interval	This refers to a scale that has numbers associated upon which mathematical operations can be performed and the magnitude of the values are respected and remain clear. That is, values may be multiplied, subtracted etc., and meaningful data are retained. However there is no zero point.	Examples include the various psychological scales based upon multiple questions summed together. A classic example is the assessment of IQ. There is debate about the acceptance of attitude scales as Interval Scales, notable examples include measures of stress or dental anxiety.
Ratio	Similar to interval scale but a zero point exists.	Celsius scale which has an absolute zero. Income level is another example.

Table 11.2

Suggested differences between quantitative and qualitative study designs

Quantitative	Issues	Qualitative
Measuring	RESEARCH PURPOSE	Understanding
Structured	RESEARCH STRATEGY	Unstructured
Static and objective	RESEARCH REALITY	Socially constructed
Hard and reliable	RESEARCH DATA	Rich and deep

certain issues or words being spoken and so present expressions of quantity. Such a distinction is therefore somewhat artificial but it permits an initial basis upon which a comparison may be made (see Table 11.2).

Some of the major designs are listed below.

Descriptive. Suitable measures may not be available for conducting a study in the researcher's area of interest. Alternatively there may be some measures that are considered appropriate but the experienced researcher may feel that, rather than relying on the opinions of others, it would be worthwhile to pinpoint the phenomenon and describe it in some detail as an account in itself, or as a backdrop to developing more formal measurements. It is important to realise that the complexity of human behaviour does not lend itself to simple numerical coding schemes. There is strength in encouraging the practitioner to write descriptive accounts of various patient interactions especially in controversial areas, such as providing both children and parents with an opportunity to have some say in the selection of a sedation method for extractions.

Observational. The scope for research into investigating human behaviour within clinical settings is huge. The use of video recordings of patient–clinician interaction in the surgery is increasing in the training of undergraduate and postgraduate dentists. Employing coding schemes to analyse both patient and dentist behaviour is highly technical and can produce vast arrays of data. The study to assess the influence of nitrous oxide in the management of disruptive children when attending the dentist relied on a moment-by-moment

methods of conducting research. However on reflection it will be clear that quantitative measures often require respondents to report their replies in verbal terms (for example, do you agree, disagree or remain neutral to this statement?) which are then converted to numbers. Researchers can sometimes become so used to transforming what respondents have said into numerical data that they forget they are dealing with people's verbal responses. Conversely qualitative methods often express their results by counting up instances of cataloguing of child and clinician behaviour (Weinstein, Domoto & Holleman 1986). However with the introduction of hand-held computers, notepads and the ever increasing size of data storage on smaller and smaller discs, the leaps in information technology achieved in the past few years make possible a more sophisticated description of patient–dentist interactions. A less overt methodology may be applied when the introduction of video or even audiotape recordings are considered intrusive.

Experimental. There is a family of designs that stems from the traditional clinical trial study in which a sample of patients are selected and randomised into an experimental group or a control group. The experimental group is given a new treatment, for example, whereas the control group is provided with standard care. A double-blind study is one in which the investigator is unaware of which patient receives the new treatment. The code is broken following the collection of all the data so that the benefits (if any) can be plotted. The management of such trials is fraught with difficulties: clear guidelines are available for the successful completion of such studies and to make the researcher aware of the possible flaws in the conduct of such studies. Single-blind is sometimes substituted for a double-blind design where the investigators cannot hide from themselves the fact that the patient receives the new intervention, for example a different type of health education programme. When randomisation is not possible quasi-experiments are conducted. For instance an evaluation of a new health promotion programme cannot be tested by randomising individual community members to different localities. The intervention is therefore run in one area and a control area is selected that matches as closely as possible (for example, in, proportion of local authority housing, car ownership or overcrowding). Interpretation of such studies is complex and in some ways requires a greater level of sophistication in research skills to determine unbiased conclusions.

Cross-sectional. This type of study tends to be descriptive and takes a 'snapshot' of the sample involved. Most surveys are cross-sectional as the work involved in following-up respondents on a second or further occasion is very time consuming and resource intensive. Useful work is completed with cross-sectional designs and researchers often test out ideas of how variables may relate to each other without making strong statements of causality.

Longitudinal. A longitudinal study involves the follow-up of the initial baseline respondents at a later date. The longer the follow-up from baseline the more likely that respondents will be lost to the study (through mobility away from the study area) and interpretation becomes more difficult. An important check is to determine who is lost to the study on follow-up, and an analysis is then conducted that shows whether the people lost to the study are different from those who are successfully followed-up. The importance of attempting longitudinal studies should not be underestimated as they do make possible firmer interpretations of causality not possible with cross-sectional designs. To illustrate with an example: if children are exposed to a traumatic first dental visit and these children are subsequently found to exhibit higher levels of disruptive behaviour in the dental surgery, then this finding would be more meaningful to understanding how experiences might cause behavioural difficulties than if the study was cross-sectional with the variable, traumatic experience and behavioural problems associated strongly at the same point in time. The cross-sectional interpretation of the results could be that the disruptive child causes the dentist to resort to management strategies that become coercive and result in a traumatic experience for the child. The cross-sectional approach therefore may produce equivocal results that encourage researchers to embark on the more ambitious longitudinal studies. The longitudinal study requires careful ethical attention, as mentioned below.

Secondary analysis. As more studies are being collected together in the literature using standard designs such as double-blind clinical trials there is a methodology which can summarise statistically the results for a number of similar studies. For instance, it may be possible to determine the extent to which psychological interventions have an influence on dental anxiety. The original paper is read and the data of the article examined carefully to derive a unit of intervention effect size, i.e. how strong was the effect of the intervention? Those studies with large effect sizes, that is, the intervention produced a strong effect, will weight the system to show an increased general effect of the factor being investigated. This review method can, for example, demonstrate the benefit of introducing presurgical information to patients about to undergo intravenous sedation. When examining for instance ten papers that have investigated this intervention the summary indices (derived from the papers) can be collated to provide an average effect size (the influence of the experimental intervention). Reviews are now published known as 'meta-analyses' which systematically aggregate the effect sizes from related studies and analyse not only the average effect size of an intervention but also determine whether certain features of an intervention tend to produce a stronger outcome. These meta-analyses have merit, particularly for discrete techniques such as school-based dental health education campaigns, as they are rigorous in their selection of studies and only include investigations where full information of the design and methods are published. Other secondary analyses are possible by applying a different statistical approach to the published tables of results, or permission may be gained to have access to the original data. New methods of data analysis or corrections to flaws in an original published paper are positive benefits of conducting secondary analyses.

Selection of measures

There are an extraordinary number of measures and assessments that may be utilised to categorise or place individuals on some continuum (known as a variable). The student can become bemused. For instance the number of self-report rating scales for dental anxiety that are currently employed in the literature are well into double figures. Even with this bewildering array of attitudinal or belief measures researchers may attempt to design their own questionnaires in order that the measures they construct exactly fit their purpose. However, the design of new measures is a notoriously difficult task to do well, and involves the commitment of a great deal of resource and effort. This work is required to ensure that the newly developed measure is clear to the respondent and possesses two important features, namely reliability and validity. A measure that is reliable is one that is internally consistent (that is, the questions which comprise the scale are associated closely together) and will give a similar result when the individual is invited to complete the measure on a subsequent occasion say a week later (Streiner & Norman 1991).

Within the behavioural sciences three main measurement techniques are employed (summarised in Box 11.2) of which there are many examples within the dental field.

OBSERVATIONS

The characteristic being assessed is assigned a category, which can then be coded into a number or described and possibly given a label. For example, disruptive behaviour of a child (see Chapter 7 for a more extensive presentation) can be simply coded into a four-category system (Frankl, Shiere & Fogels 1962) or developed into a sophisticated system requiring intensive computational support to derive indices of different types of behaviour (Weinstein et al. 1982). The use of audio and video recorders has improved our ability to collect data from observational approaches. These measures are not utilised frequently as the investment in their development is extensive. In addition the technicalities of deriving scores from assessments such as these should not be underestimated.

A less familiar method, known as ethnography, concentrates on the benefits of participant-observation. This method from the field of anthropology relies on researchers recording in a field notebook

---

BOX 11.2   TYPES OF ASSESSMENT OR
                 MEASURING TOOL

- Observation
  Field work that concentrates on the
  collection of notes of behaviours,
  conversations, results of meetings,
  clinical sessions or home visits.
  Coding of behaviour from in vivo
  scenarios e.g. in the surgery, or from
  videotape.
- Interviews
  Open-ended interviews are held without
  present time limits or agendas according
  to content. Some topics may be
  determined prior to interviewing. Used
  when sensitive issues are discussed e.g.
  sexual practices and illicit drug usage,
  and the researcher wishes to give free
  rein to the participant in the research.
  Closed or structured interviewing has a
  firm format to adhere to and produces
  data that are often easier to analyse,
  although the stronger framework can be
  constricting.
- Standardised questionnaires
  Checklists can be compiled which are
  simple to complete and produce rapid
  data collection. Requires heavy
  investment to assess validity of the
  replies.
- Rating scales are similar to checklists but
  provide the respondent with an
  opportunity to give a ranking to their
  reply. Can become sophisticated in their
  design and technical in their
  interpretation (the area is termed
  psychometrics).

---

every significant event that is witnessed when amongst the group they wish to study. The reactions of the researchers to events around them are noted. The ethnographer researcher will spend many hours, days or weeks in the company of the people he is researching so as to 'live' like them. Data may be contained in field notebooks, audiocassette tapes and photographs, although the relationship of the researcher to this data is not as independent observer but rather as someone who tries to tell a story from the view of the people being studied. An example of this method has been applied to dentistry (Nettleton 1986).

INTERVIEWS

The researcher speaks to an individual and attempts to understand the replies offered – at first hand the interview appears simple, almost trivial in its ability to gain useful data. However the social scientist relies strongly on this technique to develop new areas of enquiry and topics which are not amenable to formal testing and assessment. A new area has been the public's response to HIV and the lack of suitable measures to assess knowledge and attitudes towards HIV infection and those who have HIV. The various beliefs held by individuals – both staff and patients – were not easily amenable to formal pencil and paper questionnaires and could only be tapped by in-depth discussion. From in-depth interviewing validity is regarded as superior as the individual being questioned can reply unfettered by supplied schemes of response such as a rating scale. However, whether an individual would reply to a question in the same way on a different occasion (that is, raising the issue of reliability) is an important one and is answered by the interviewer stating that the conditions were different under interviewing on both occasions and hence reliability is not a central issue with this form of data collection. In order to ensure a coherent system of assessment without stifling patient-centred responses, the patient can be interviewed in depth with further interviews completed in a different setting – thus avoiding, for example, the propensity to become nervous when visiting the dentist, a factor which may have been apparent in the previous interview.

QUESTIONNAIRES

This method of data collection is popular and growing in usage. Patients' feelings, attitudes and beliefs are amenable to recording either through verbatim written responses, or more commonly with rating scales and tick boxes. The simple rating scale can be given a number according to the answer given by the respondent (e.g. 1 = strongly agree, 2 = agree, 3 = undecided, 4 = disagree, 5 = strongly disagree). These coding schemes are relatively easy to apply and produce meaningful data. However care has to be taken as the simple tick box response can be illusory and various validity checks are required to assist in interpretation. Researchers in the dental field searching for a suitable questionnaire are encouraged to use already developed scales (such as the Dental Anxiety Scale) to which comparisons can be made rather than developing 'in-house' versions.

In summary, the selection of a measure or set of measures can be one of the most difficult tasks for the researcher. A measure may not exist for the purposes of the study you wish to conduct. This may necessitate the development of a new scale or selection of a less than optimal measure. Measures should possess reliability and validity.

Reliability refers to the degree to which a measure will give the same result if repeated. Two types of reliability are commonly quoted (Streiner & Norman 1991). First, *test-retest reliability* refers to the association between two administrations of the measure. The difficulty in interpreting these reliability coefficients (ranging from 0 to 1, where 1 is perfect reliability and 0 shows none) is to judge what is a suitable period to leave between the two testings. Too short a duration and the patient will remember his previous response, too long a duration and the construct, – the thing being measured – will have changed either because the individual has matured or because some intervening variable has altered the measure. The second type of reliability is known as *internal consistency*, and refers to the degree that the items (e.g. ratings or question responses) that constitute the measure relate to each other. Internal consistency can only be assessed if the measure consists of more than one single element. The concept is analogous to using a ruler to measure a piece of string not just once but, for example, four times. The four measures should relate well together but may not agree entirely due to some error of measurement. Similarly, assessments in social science are usually error prone, but this can be managed by introducing a number of related questions which will provide a stronger picture of the construct that the

study is attempting to tap. This strategy is commonly adopted in questionnaire-based surveys and experiments trying to assess social science variables such as attitudes and beliefs.

Validity is an important concept in measurement selection and interpretation of results. The term validity refers to the extent that the measure utilised reflects what was intended, so that a measure of dental pain, for instance, should give the researcher a close estimate of the pain experienced by the patient. Testing whether a measure is valid is not straightforward and requires some ingenuity. One method is to approach others (say experts) and poll whether they consider the measure to reflect what it is supposed to. Streiner (Streiner & Norman 1991) refers to this as the 'malt whisky' validity rather the more familiar '*content validity*'. He refers to the situation in which a researcher asks a group of academic friends to endorse the newly developed measure in return for a gift!

A second method is to test the measure against a more familiar 'gold standard'. This method is known as *criterion validity*. Unfortunately, it tends to beg the question: why design a new measure in the first place, other than the possibility that the new measure may be reduced in size, or simplified? Therefore criterion validity is not sufficient.

A third method, known as *construct validity*, is to formulate what relationship your new measure will have with other constructs. For example, a new measure of self-reported pain will be expected to relate closely to the respondent's reports of anxiety and use of painkillers. In addition the pain measure is not likely to relate closely to a patient's intelligence level (unless the questionnaire is complexly worded) or to income, and a network of relationships can therefore be established with additional variables that flesh out a profile of the new measure. An interesting consequence of this form of validity is that the measure that is developed will only be as good as the theory upon which it is based.

Validity is harder to achieve than reliability. The researcher may be lulled into a false sense of security with a measure showing strong reliability, only to find with further work that the new measure was assessing some other feature. Those who specialise in qualitative research would state that the effort to demonstrate reliability is misplaced and that the vital commodity is the validity of the measurement.

The search for reliability and validity from a qualitative perspective is not conducted in ways accepted by quantitative researchers. Qualitative researchers would be suspicious of the estimates of validity that are quoted for quantitative measures in the literature. The manner in which knowledge is acquired (referred to as epistemology) does not lend itself to the formal traditional systems employed by quantitative proponents. The issue of validity is of central importance to qualitative researchers and their methods attempt to draw on the respondent's beliefs and opinions without placing a 'straightjacket' on the individual. Attention to assessing validity is important to the qualitative researcher (Smith 1996 p 192) and methods employed are listed here.

Internal coherence. The data should present clear arguments and be able to explain ambiguities and contradictory evidence that arises. The researcher should have outlined possible alternative explanations and given coherent reasons for accepting their preferred formulation.

Presentation of evidence. There should be sufficient raw data presented to enable readers to perform a simple analysis for themselves and derive identical or at least similar findings. Space restrictions in a report or journal may prevent sufficient material for the researcher to satisfy this validation check. It may be possible without breaking participants' confidentiality to offer transcripts to interested readers to share the material and encourage an openness to reinterpretation.

Independent audit. The material collected in the study (transcripts, field notes and diaries for example) can be vetted by an independent researcher, who can provide evidence to support the explanatory stance adopted by the original researcher.

Triangulation. In order to demonstrate the validity of a method such as interviewing and relying on transcripts, the researcher may adopt additional methods to support the findings obtained by the initial and preferred

method. An example from the field of health needs assessment is using a WHO derived approach known as 'rapid appraisal' where a locality is focused on to identify the community priorities with regard to health and health services, and includes interviewing prominent community 'experts' (Ong et al. 1991). In order to check for potential interviewer bias one of the methods incorporated was to introduce an observation phase (that is, walking around the locality looking for evidence and therefore behaving like an ethnographer) and a library phase (searching widely for documents that tended to support the transcript findings, thereby demonstrating the skills of an archivist). Findings reported from a study in Liverpool that used this technique illustrate such a validation method. The transcripts identified asthma as a key problem in young children, and observations made when visiting nurseries as to the number of children carrying inhalers or 'puffers' confirmed this. In addition the records of local pharmacists showed an above-average distribution of inhalers compared with regional averages.

Selection of an appropriate sample

Selecting a sample requires careful consideration whatever design you choose. It is highly unlikely that the researcher can collect data from every member of the public that comprise the target group. It is accepted therefore that a proportion of the whole population is drawn, known as a sample. Although these terms have specific definitions for experimenters and survey designers the concept of obtaining a sample is readily appreciated.

Random samples. There are recognised sampling schemes which are employed for different purposes; the most commonly referred to sampling strategy is randomised. As the name suggests, individuals are selected from a specified group in a fashion in which the selection of any one individual is based purely on chance. In practice these conditions are not always easily achieved, hence a description of how the participants were selected is important to include in any write up. A related area of concern is representativeness. It is hoped that a randomly selected sample will closely represent the actual characteristics of the total population of the group under study. The degree of representiveness will however also be dependent on how large a sample is being drawn. A small sample will derive a group description (say a mean or average value) that does not represent well the group being investigated. Complex sampling strategies (such as stratified sampling) are available which can assist representativeness. *Convenience sampling.* Where random sampling is impossible or highly expensive a form of sampling known as convenience sampling is practised – as its name suggests this is a method whereby individuals are drawn without recourse to randomisation but through simple membership at a point in time when the researcher wishes to conduct their study. An example of a convenience sample may be to select the first 100 adults encountered in the High Street to ask them about a recent health promotion campaign.

WRITING A PROTOCOL

An important stage in starting research is the writing of a protocol. This document states the background to the proposed research, its aims and objectives, its hypotheses expressed formally as null hypotheses ('this new treatment will not demonstrate an improvement in the quality of life of the patient') or simply as a research question ('To what extent will patients' quality of life improve from receipt of the new treatment?'). The methods need to be detailed simply and clearly under headings similar to these: materials, measures, sample, procedure. A section on the statistical treatment or handling of the data is required, and some statement of how the results will be disseminated. Key references need to be listed in full at the end of the document, with copies of the interview schedule, questionnaire, data proforma, observation sheet etc., attached. It is an excellent

idea to find an experienced colleague or supervisor to read the protocol before submission to the ethical committee.

ETHICAL APPROVAL

Before starting a study involving participants the Local Ethical Committee (LOC) must be approached and a protocol supplied to the chair for approval. There are strict guidelines to which the LOC can advise the researcher to adhere. A discussion with the LOC is important if issues are potentially ambiguous, – for example should consent to take part in a proposed study involving adolescents be invited from both parent and young person? LOCs will expect a reason for the study to be conducted, its possible benefits (for example, improved understanding or increase in knowledge). A consent form requiring the participant's signature – with a statement that he or she is free to refuse to take part without prejudice to treatment or services received – must be completed if the study involves patients.

PILOT WORK

Most studies will benefit from conducting a pilot study, and sometimes more than one is required. The purpose of this pilot is to test the methods and administration of the study. The collection of data is dependent on a variety of procedures, for example the researcher has to locate the sample, gain consent, conduct the interview or administer the questionnaire and make observations. Many elements of this may not go to plan and so the study design may require adjustments. Many studies require modification as a result of difficulties in identifying suitable participants. This is particularly the case with clinically related projects where a certain number of people are required to fit specified criteria (inclusion or exclusion). It is often the case that as soon as a study is planned to investigate a particular patient group, that particular group becomes a rarity. The pilot study can also be considered a training period for the researcher to become more confident with the methodology, observation scheme, interview schedule or the people under investigation. If changes are made to the pilot study as a result, such as a modification to the measures employed, then the researcher must re-examine the original research question(s) and objectives to ascertain if the study itself is dramatically changed. Pilot studies inevitably improve the research and are strongly recommended, even if the data collected are not analysed extensively.

Main study

When the main study is embarked upon then the procedures should remain the same throughout. This is especially true of clinical trial experiments. With in-depth interviewing however, each interview may adopt different procedures of prompting and the direction of the interview may alter according to the content that is collected from the participant. Even with the more flexible approach required of the in-depth interview, it is still imperative to follow the methods employed for that technique, and to note any change or violation of the process of conducting the research. For instance, the researcher should note carefully when interviewing if there is an interruption, or if the participant requires another person to be present (such as a friend or parent) for support. Changes may have to be made to the main study design should unforeseeable circumstances intervene. There are many examples of changes to health services from government or health authority, changes to the law, withdrawal of certain forms of treatment or drug therapy that preclude the maintenance of the study procedure. This is frustrating for the researcher, however it is unlikely to completely invalidate the study as there is always some benefit from embarking on a study and collecting data.

Security of data

All data collected must be stored securely to ensure confidentiality and prevent valuable loss of information. If data is to be stored on computer (either in numerical form as codes from a questionnaire or in words verbatim from open-ended interviews)

then care must be made to register it under the Data Protection Act. Most higher education establishments and health organisations have arrangements locally for storing data that will be permitted under the Act. Unless strictly necessary it is not good practice to collect data that has names and addresses of participants on computer even if secured under file password protection. Longitudinal study designs that collect data from the same set of individuals to investigate change in a set of designated variables such as dental health indices and patient perceptions of need for treatment will require code numbers to ensure a matching of their data from one instance of data collection to the next. For instance a two-year study collecting, say, 100 individuals' attitudes to visiting the dentist will follow what is known as this 'cohort' of 100 over the two years and match together the individuals' replies. This method is one way of determining change in attitudes and behaviour over time and how each may have an influence on the other.

Analysis of results

One of the most interesting tasks for the researcher is the analysis of the collected data. Whether the data is in the form of words or numbers will determine how it is treated. Researchers are often required to enter their data onto computer in some form. Qualitative researchers who may collect large quantities of verbal material from interviews may enter their data in a word-processor file before importing the statements into a specialist computer program which can assist in categorising the statements. Quantitative data can be entered into spreadsheet or database computer applications or fed directly into statistical programs. Examples of packaged statistical software include Minitab™ which is a good program for learning statistical routines. The Statistical Package for the Social Sciences (SPSS), in its various versions, is a popular and widespread program for survey and experimental data sets, and other packages include SAS, SYSTAT and BMDP. A popular package for dental survey work is EPINFO. The statistical analysis of data is an important aid in determining whether your predictions have been confirmed. Studies can be categorised into those that are interested in the relationship between the variables that have been collected, such as whether attitudes are associated with behaviour, and those that concentrate on whether one group has a higher or lower level on an entity than the other group. Statistical approaches are available for example to ascertain whether people without teeth are more anxious than those with teeth.

REPORT WRITING

A standard structure for producing a report is shown in Box 11.3. A report should inform the reader why the study was done and why the methods chosen appeared to the researcher the best way of achieving the aims. It will become obvious to the individual approaching research for the first time that the variety of methods and approaches are considerable. A great many of the decisions to be taken can be made with the help of a supervisor and by reading widely in the area of interest as well as in the large number of research method books now available. However the actual 'doing' of the research is a crucial learning process which should be reflected in the report. The reader is interested not only in the results and conclusions but also in what difficulties were encountered and how the study could be improved. This level of description allows the reader to learn of potential pitfalls and make attempts to approach the field of study either from a different direction or adopting some of the recommended improvements building upon the previously reported work.

PUBLICATION

The researcher's responsibility is to publish the results of studies that are conducted so that they are in the public domain and available to a readership that can appreciate the work. The opportunities for getting your work into print have never been greater, with an explosion of academic and professional journals; putting material 'on the Web' is a further avenue likely to gain popularity especially because of its rapid production and ease of access. Some organisations have publications specifically for the novice researcher which are

---

BOX 11.3   TRADITIONAL STRUCTURE FOR
WRITING A REPORT

- Title
- Background or introduction
- Aims and objectives
- Methods
    Measures (formal questionnaire) or data collection technique such as audiotape recording or detailed case/field notes
    Participants
    Procedure
    Statistical analyses where appropriate
    Results
    Present basic description of data
    Present interpretative analyses
- Discussion
    Main findings from results section: refer to past literature to determine if consistent findings have been found
    Limitations of study and cautionary notes on interpretations
    Future work required
- Conclusions and recommendations
- References
- Executive summary or abstract (may go at start of report).

---

worth exploring as they are sympathetic to the first time writer. Another avenue is to team up with an experienced writer of papers (such as a supervisor) and offer to complete a draft for their editing. Patience and persistence are required when submitting to journals.

References

Frankl S N, Shiere F R, Fogels H R 1962 Should the parent remain with the child in the dental operatory? Journal of Dentistry for Children 29:150–163

Hammersley M 1996 The relationship between qualitative and quantitative research: paradigm loyalty versus methodological eclecticism. In: Richardson J (ed.) Handbook of qualitative research methods for psychology and the social sciences. Leicester: BPS Books

Nettleton S 1986 Understanding dental health beliefs: an introduction to ethnography. British Dental Journal 161:145–147

Ong B N, Humphris G M, Annett H, Rifkin S 1991 Rapid appraisal in an urban setting, an example from the developed world. Social Science and Medicine 32:909–915

Smith J 1996 Evolving issues for qualitative psychology. In: Richardson J (ed.) Handbook of qualitative research methods for psychology and the social sciences. Leicester: BPS Books

Streiner D, Norman G 1991 Health measurement scales: a practical guide to their development and use. Oxford: Oxford University Press

Weinstein P, Domato P, Holleman E 1986 The use of nitrous oxide in the treatment of children: results of a controlled study. Journal of the American Dental Association 112:325–321

Weinstein P, Getz T, Ratener P, Domato P 1982 The effect of dentists' behaviors on fear-related behaviors in children. Journal of the American Dental Association 104:32–38

Index